Jesse's Magic Plate

BY DONNA DAUN LESTER

ILLUSTRATED BY CHRISTINA KRATI

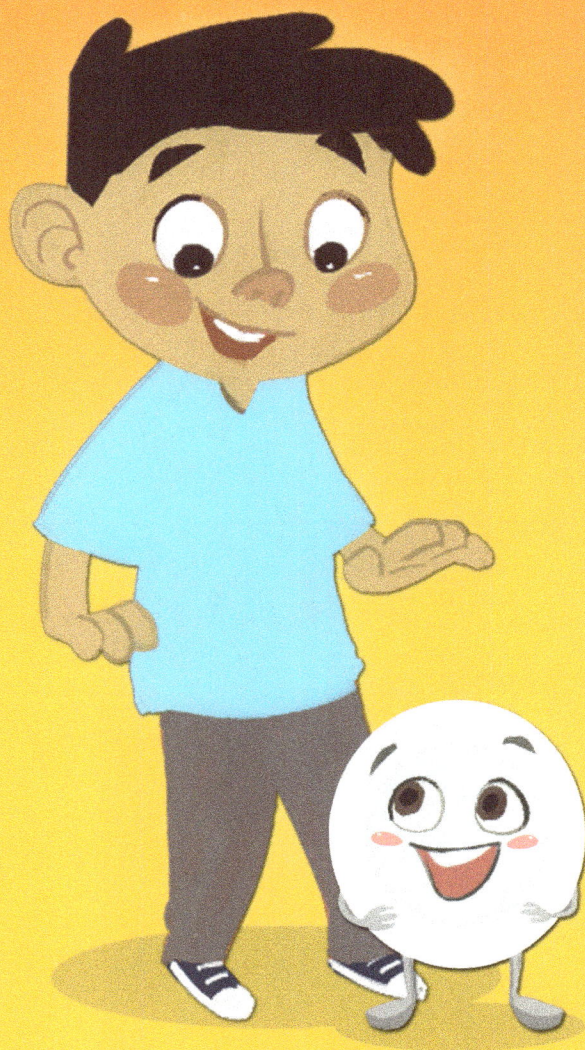

For

Katherine Bell and Victoria Daun

...my Magic Plate young visionaries

DDL

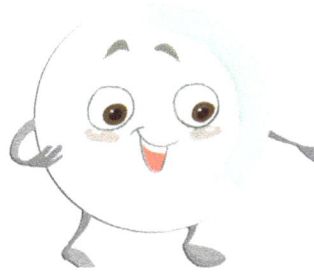

TABLE OF CONTENTS

Author's Note
Message from the Author

PART ONE

PART TWO

Acknowledgements
About the Author and Illustrator

AUTHOR'S NOTE

It is very important to speak with your doctor before making any changes to your or a child's diet or level of exercise. Neither Nutrition Network Publishers Inc., nor the author, can be held responsible for illness (including food allergies), or any other health issues that may result from anyone trying anything described in this book.

Published in the United States of America by
Nutrition Network Publishers Inc.

jessesmagicplate.com

Publisher's Cataloging-in-Publication data

Lester, Donna Daun.
    Jesse's magic plate / by Donna Daun Lester ; story illustration by Christina Krati.

    p. cm.
    ISBN 978-0-9898633-4-6 (pbk.)
    ISBN 978-0-9898633-1-5 (Hardcover)
    ISBN 978-0-9898633-0-8 (pbk.)

    Summary : Jesse encounters a Magic Plate that teaches him how to eat healthfully, and the importance of good nutrition and exercise for optimal health.

[1. Nutrition --Fiction. 2. Diet --Fiction. 3. Health --Fiction. 4. Food --Fiction. 5. Exercise --Fiction.]
I. Krati, Christina. II. Title.

PZ7.L562845 Je 2014
[E] --dc23   2013915487

First Edition
Printed in the United States of America

MESSAGE FROM THE AUTHOR

Much of my inspiration for *Jesse's Magic Plate* came from my use, as a nutrition educator, of the USDA MyPlate food guidance system. MyPlate is a nutrition education initiative developed to promote important nutrition recommendations from the US Dietary Guidelines for Americans.

I am a great fan of MyPlate, and I encourage everyone to visit <u>choosemyplate.gov</u>. There, you'll be able to view healthful meal plans for each age group, find recipes, and learn a great deal about nutrition. In the Super-Tracker section, you can track and analyze your daily intake, analyze your own recipes, and more.

Did you know that foods contain even more nutrients than those listed on the Nutrition Facts label? Check out the MyPlate Super-Tracker Food-A-Pedia section where you can obtain and compare complete nutrition information for thousands of foods. While there, be sure to sign up for daily nutrition email updates!

I believe that healthful foods *do* have super-natural powers. They are so much more than foods. They are marvelous, delicious gifts from Mother Nature, super-powered with essential nutrients that we all need to be healthy and strong. When one considers that researchers have identified more than 50 essential nutrients, it seems miraculous that nature has provided all we need. All we have to do is eat healthfully!

Nature gave us even more. For example, substances such as the antioxidants and phytonutrients in healthy foods help to protect us against various diseases. Super-natural power foods can even provide health benefits above and beyond that of being well nourished!

I love the idea that we can magically transform an ordinary plate into a Magic Plate, just by filling it with, and eating the correct amounts of, healthy foods.

In *Jesse's Magic Plate*, the plate needs exercise, just as people do. Exercise is a vital component of good health, and the program Let's Move! is a wonderful initiative in support of exercise for children. You can find out more by visiting <u>letsmove.gov</u>. Let's Move! is dedicated to solving the challenge of childhood obesity, so that children born today will grow up healthy and be able to pursue their dreams.

I hope you enjoy the story of *Jesse's Magic Plate* and that it will inspire you to be the best you can be, for your health, and for the health of those you love.

Donna Daun Lester, MA, RDN, CDN

PART ONE

1

TAKE ME HOME

Like most kids, Jesse never paid any attention to plates. As long as he could put food on them, he thought one plate was the same as the next.

But Jesse was in for a big surprise!

He was about to learn that wonderful treasures can be found in the most unexpected places.

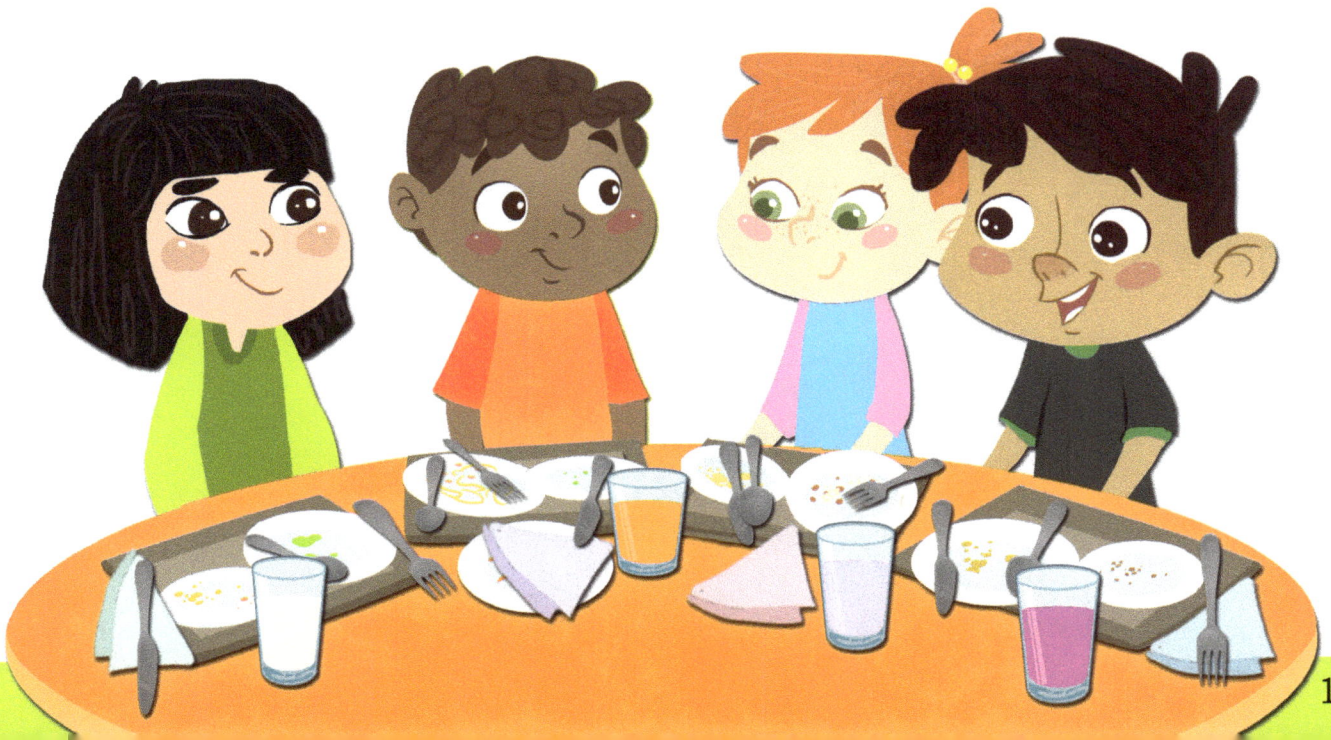

One day, Jesse's mom brought him to a secondhand store.

Jesse enjoyed seeing all kinds of things that had once belonged to other people.

As Jesse walked around, he saw some dishes.

"Pssst!"

Was that a sound he heard?

Jesse looked, but there was no one nearby.

Jesse turned away, but heard the sound again, even louder.

"PSSST!"

Jesse searched once more, then suddenly stopped.

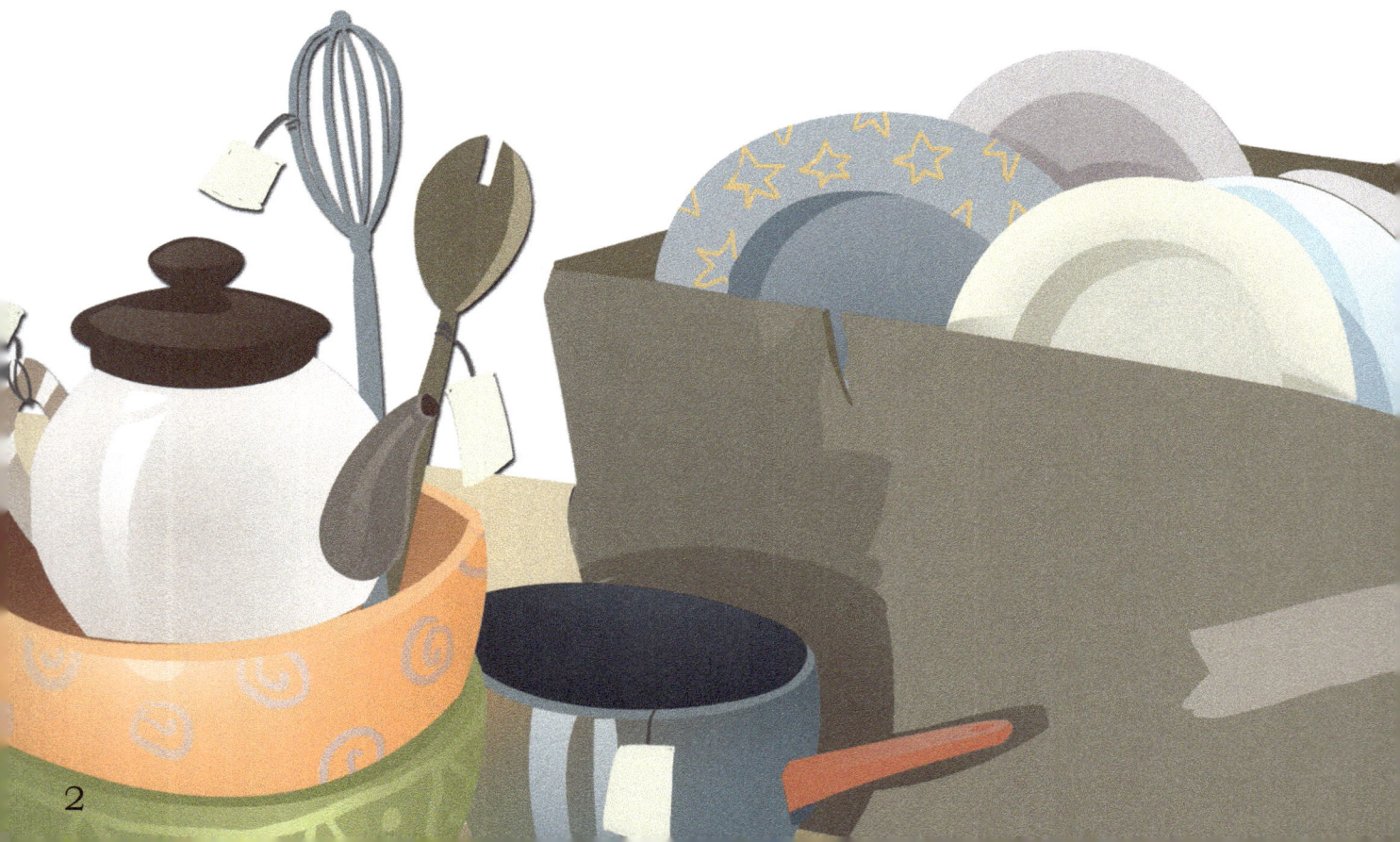

He could hardly believe his eyes. A funny-looking white plate was standing up and waving at him!

It had bright round eyes, arms made of forks, legs made of spoons, and a big cheerful smile.

"Wow, a toy plate!" Jesse shouted as he walked closer.

"Shh!" whispered the plate. "I'm not a toy. I'm alive!"

"You can't be," whispered Jesse. "Plates aren't alive!"

"Yes, I *am*," whispered the plate. "I'm a Magic Plate and I need your help!"

Jesse didn't believe that *any* plate could be magical, but he decided to pretend that he did. He was curious about how he could help.

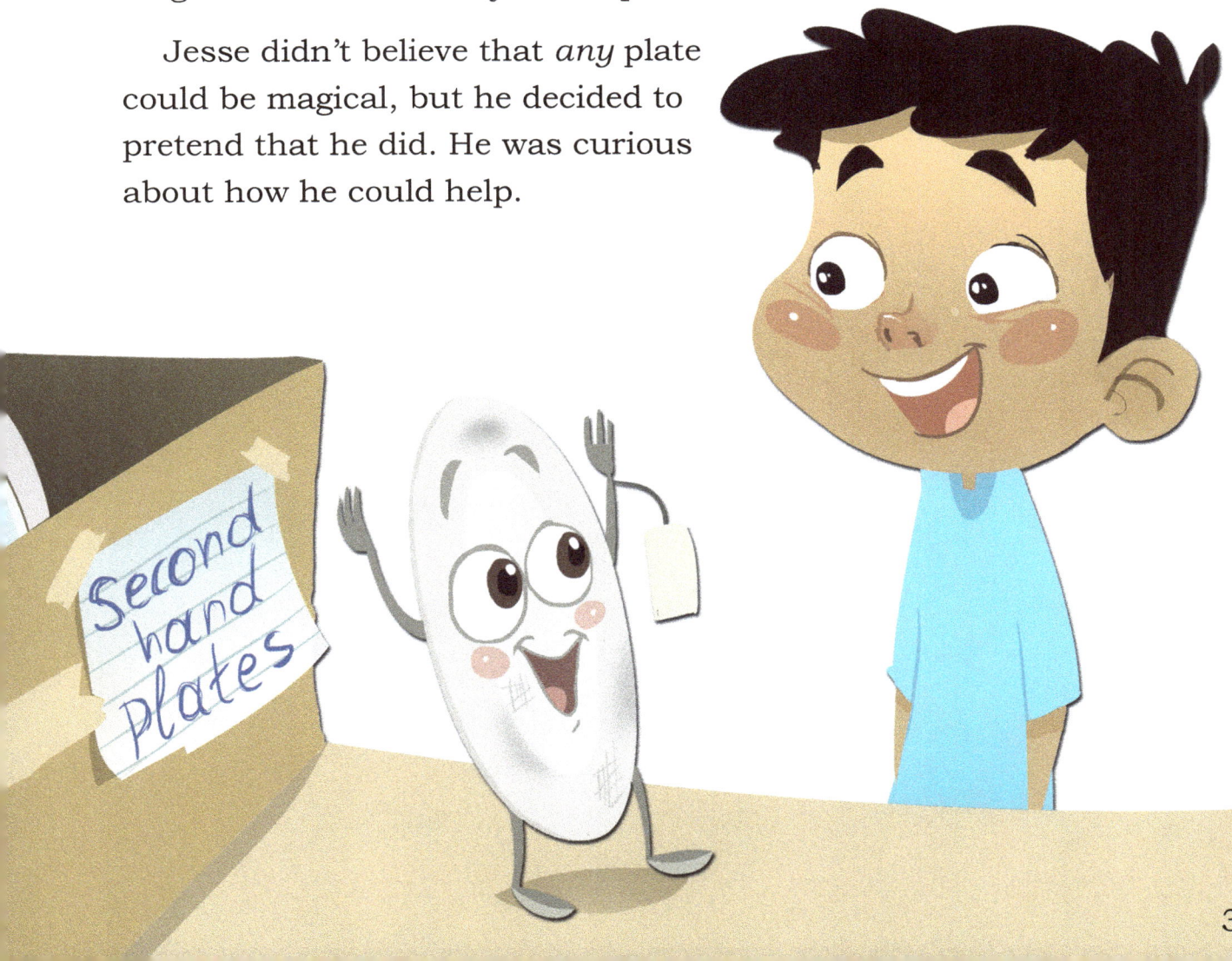

Second hand plates

"What kind of help do you need?" Jesse asked.

"I want to go home with you," the plate said.

"Why?" Jesse asked.

The plate explained that it used to live with a family that treasured it, but when the children grew up, they forgot how special the plate was, and they gave it to the secondhand store.

"I'm lonely," said the plate. "I want to have friends again, but grown-ups don't want to buy me. I'm a little worn out, so they think I'm junk. I've been wishing all this time for a child to come and take me home. I'm so glad you're here, Jesse!"

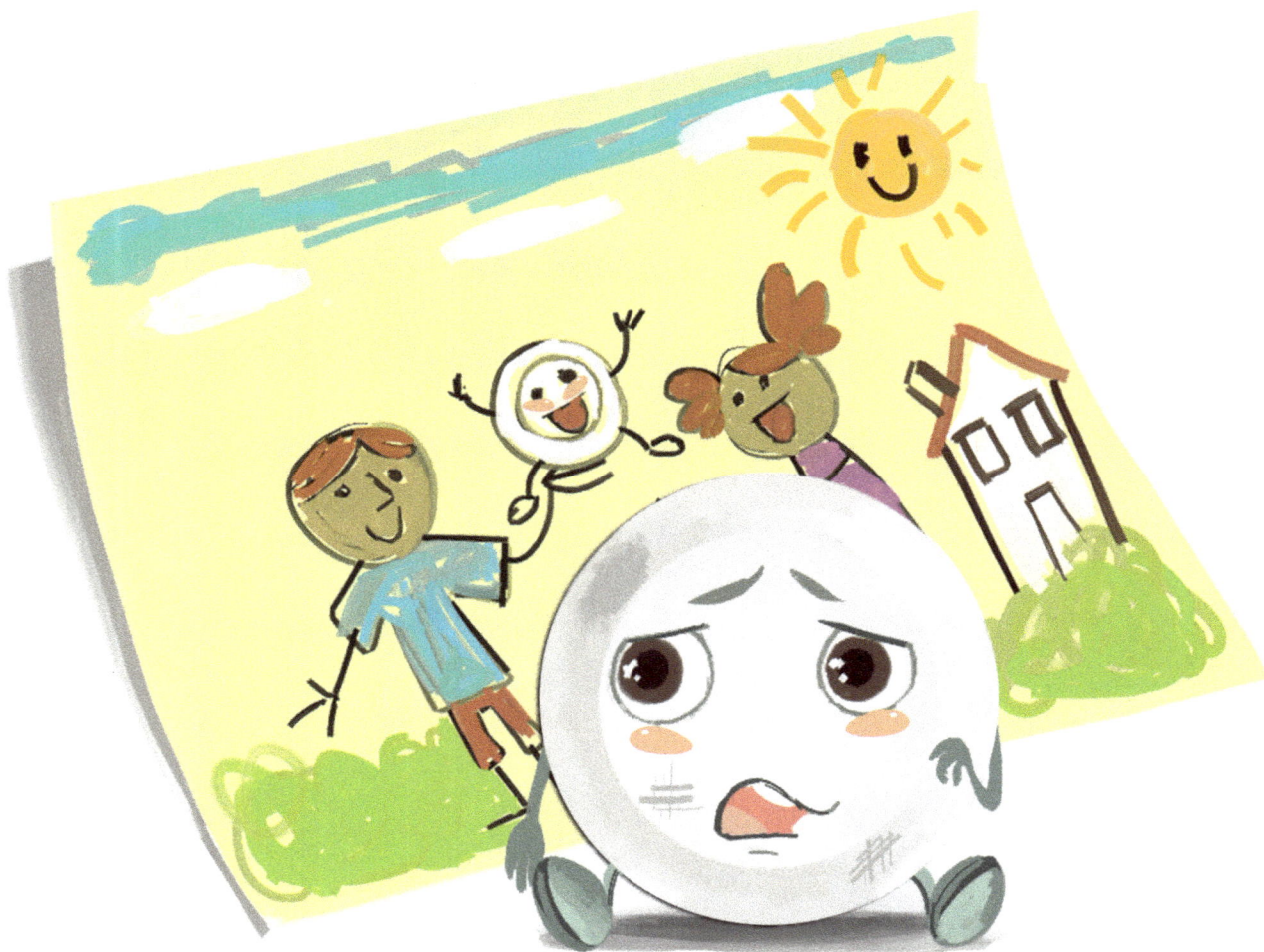

"How do you know my name?" Jesse asked the plate.

"I told you," said the plate, "I'm a Magic Plate."

Jesse was starting to believe the plate.

"I can't just take you home with me," Jesse told the plate. "I'd have to buy you, and I don't have any money."

"Please ask your mom," begged the plate. "I promise, you'll be so glad to have me."

Jesse thought for a moment. "All right, I'll try," he said. "But I think you should pretend to be a regular plate so you don't scare my mom."

"Okay!" said the plate, as it laid down flat and behaved its very plate best.

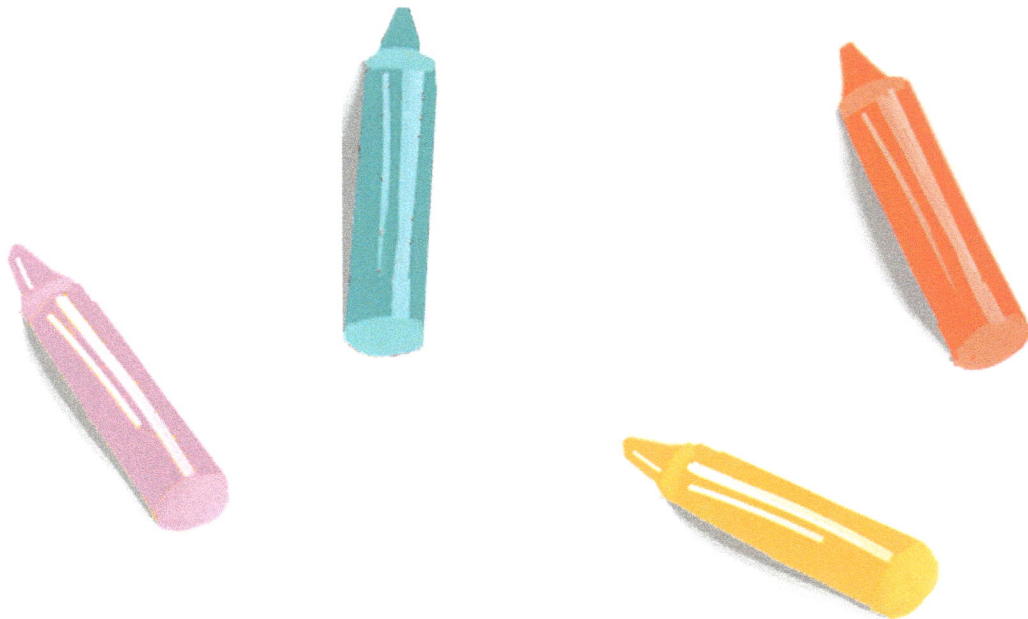

Jesse picked up the plate and carried it over to his mom.

"Mom, can we please buy this plate?" asked Jesse.

"Why?" his mom asked. "We have so many plates at home."

"Well,...I just like it," said Jesse.

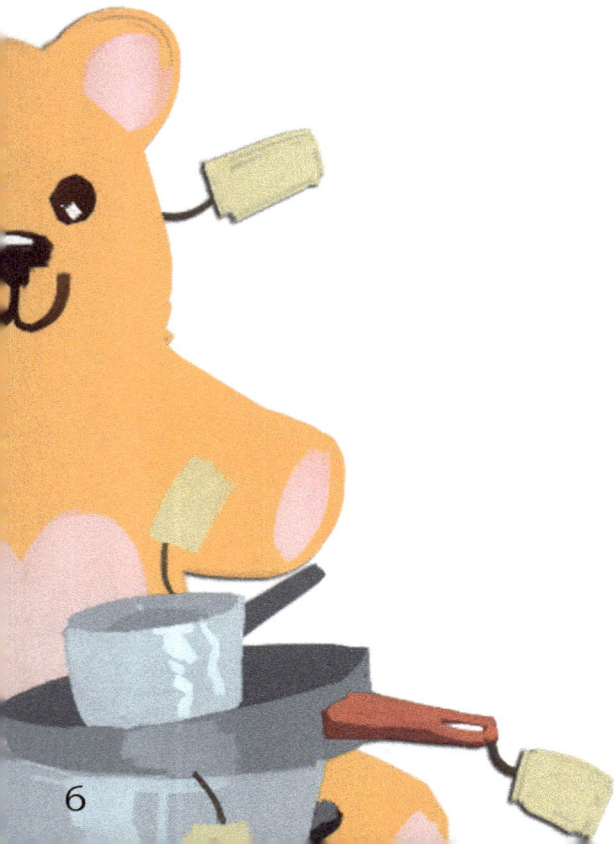

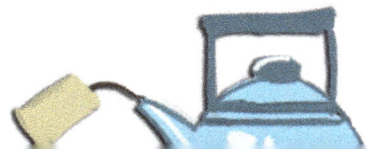

Jesse's mom turned to the store clerk. "How much does this plate cost?" she asked.

"Oh, there's no charge for that plate," said the clerk. "You are welcome to have it. It's an old children's plate and no one seems to want it. I'm glad we won't have to throw it away."

Hearing this, the little plate blushed and felt very embarrassed.

Jesse felt bad for the little plate, and decided he was glad he was going to help.

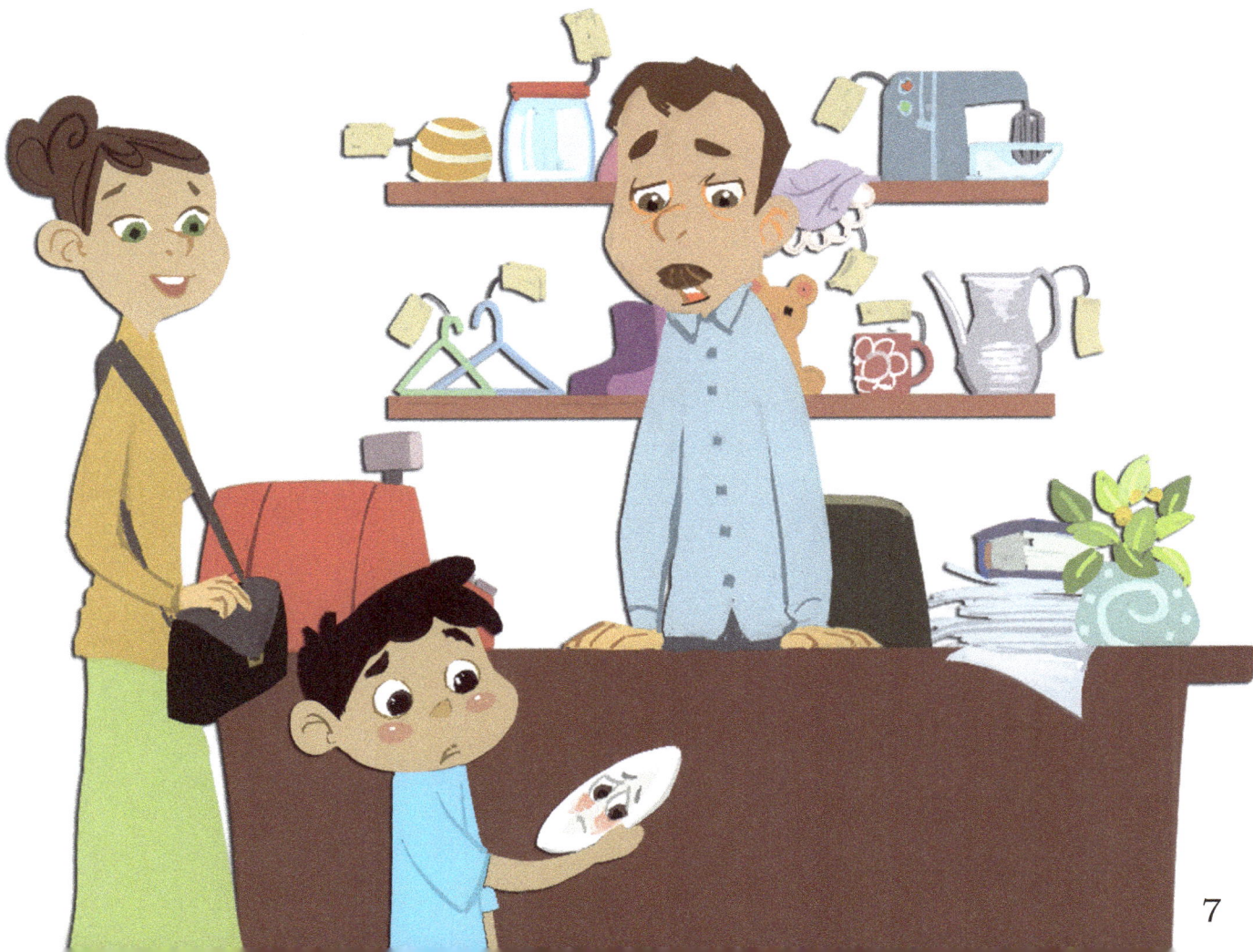

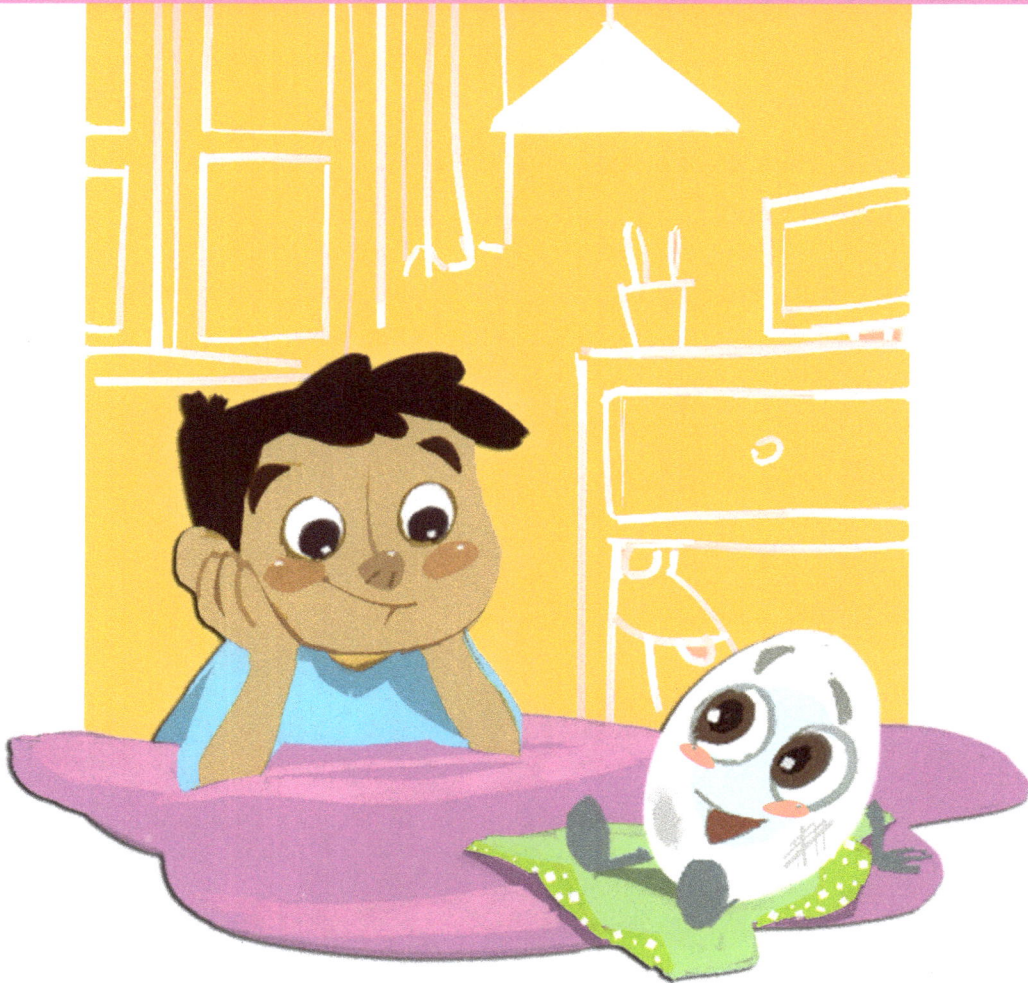

Back home, Jesse carried the plate up to his room and unwrapped it. The plate stood up, stretched its fork arms wide, and settled down with a smile.

"It feels so nice to be back in a home," the plate said, looking around.

"Please remember to act like a regular plate in front of my mom," Jesse reminded the plate.

"Don't worry, I know what to do!" said the plate, as it did its very best to lie flat all afternoon while Jesse played in his room.

2

THE BEST WE CAN BE

When Jesse's mom called him for dinner, the plate stood up.

"Where are you going?" Jesse asked the plate.

"Aren't you going to take me to dinner with you?" the plate asked.

"Why would I do that?" asked Jesse.

"Why not?" asked the plate. "Plates get hungry too! Besides, children always feed me. That's how I get to be the best I can be."

"The best you can be?" asked Jesse. "You're just a plate!"

"No one is *just anything*," said the plate. "*Any* of us can be our best if we want to badly enough, even plates!"

"Come on," said Jesse. "How can you be better than a plate?"

"It has to do with foods," said the plate. "There are things about foods that many grown-ups know, but most kids don't."

"Like what?" Jesse asked, eagerly.

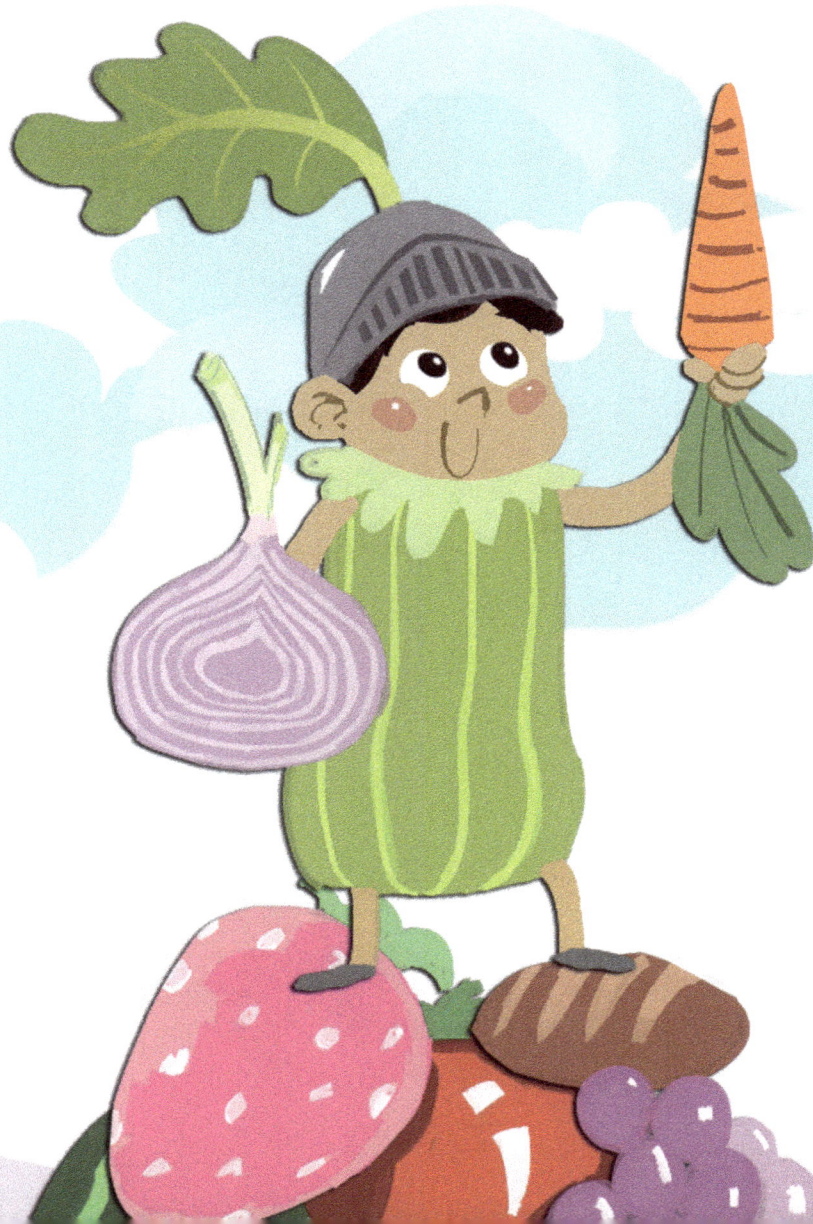

"There are foods that have super-natural powers," the plate said.

"Super-natural powers?" Jesse repeated.

"That's right," said the plate. "Nature gave its foods super-natural powers to keep us healthy and strong. People who eat those foods are the best they can be, and so are their plates."

"Do you expect me to believe that there are foods with super-natural powers?" Jesse asked the plate.

"Yes," the plate said, "and I can teach you all about it. Magic Plates are here to teach people, especially kids."

"There are other Magic Plates?" asked Jesse.

"Of course!" said the plate. "There are many of us. We're all on the lookout for super-natural power foods so people can be their very best."

"Well, I'm not sure I believe this," said Jesse, "but I could use some magic in my life right now. Our softball team is on a losing streak, and my grades need all the help they can get."

"That's where I come in!" said the plate, feeling proud to be helpful again, as it went downstairs to dinner with Jesse.

3

SUPER-NATURAL POWER FOODS

At dinner, Jesse ate chicken, but didn't want to eat carrots.

"Would you like some pasta?" Jesse's mom asked.

"Sure," Jesse replied.

For dessert, Jesse's mom offered him some strawberries, but Jesse said, "No thanks. May I have some ice cream instead?"

Jesse hoped that his plate was enjoying dinner as much as he was.

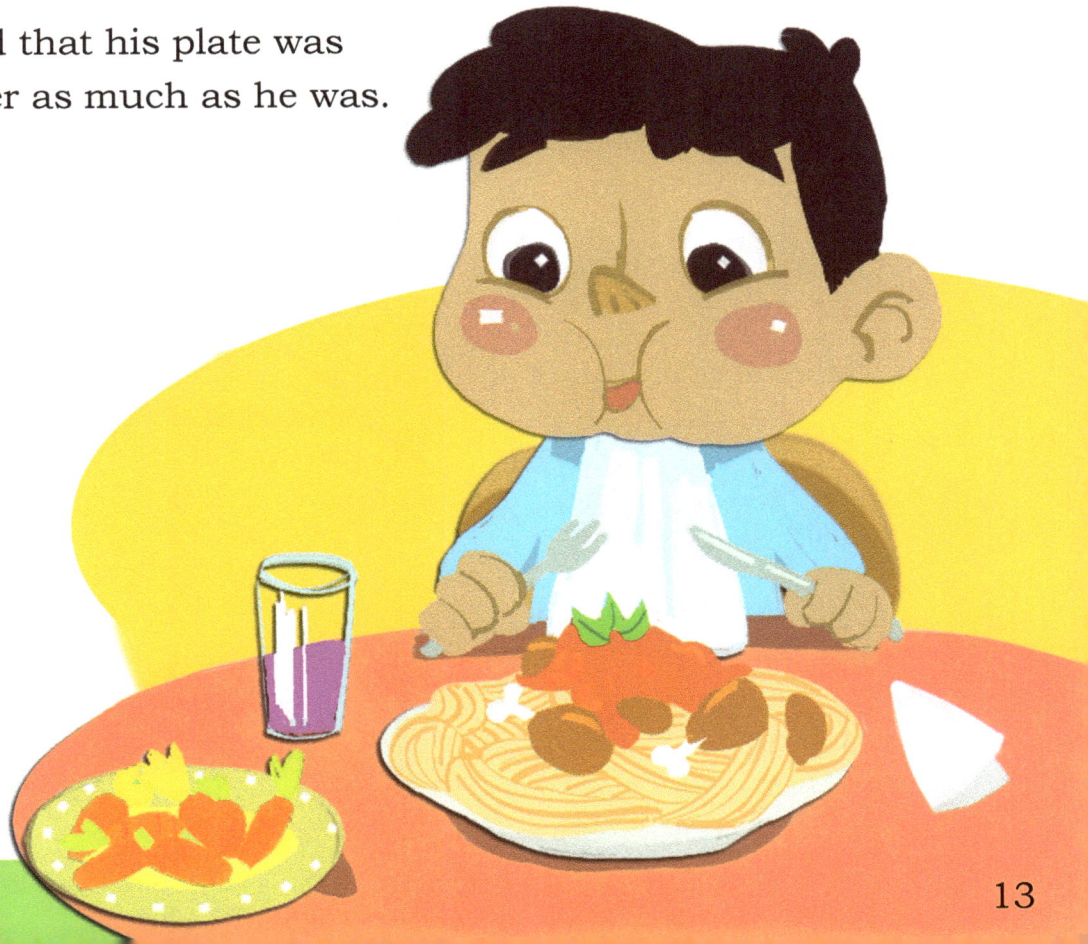

After dinner, Jesse brought the plate back up to his room.

"You did great, Jesse!" said the plate. "The chicken and pasta were delicious. Chicken is one of the protein power foods. Foods like fish and beans are, too. Protein foods help to keep our muscles strong and help us grow..."

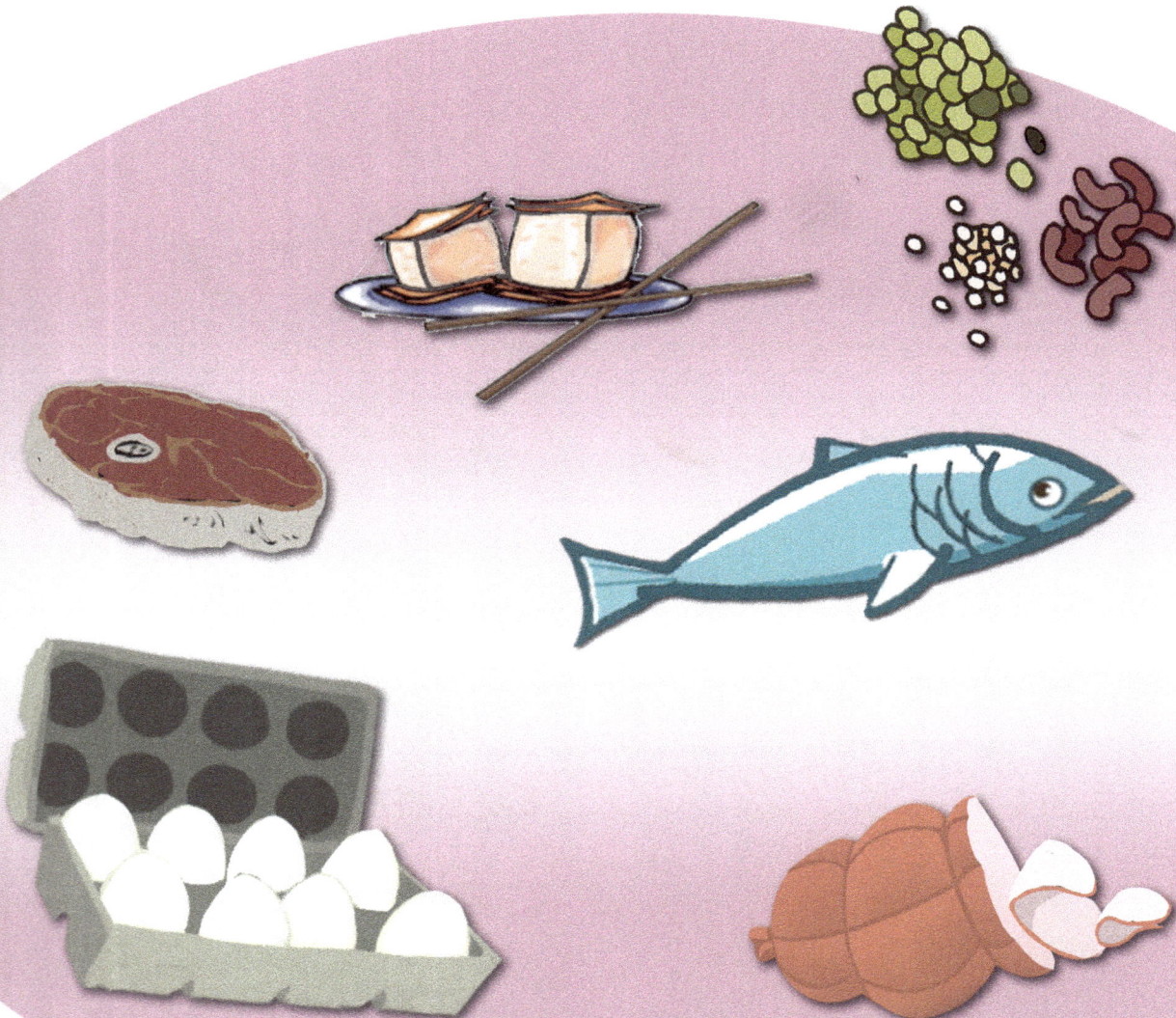

(For more information about Protein Foods, turn to page 83)

"Wait a minute," said Jesse. "What muscles do *you* have?"

"How do you think I get around?" asked the plate. "Magic Plates need strong muscles and exercise to stay active and healthy, just like people do. Besides, I like to stay in shape."

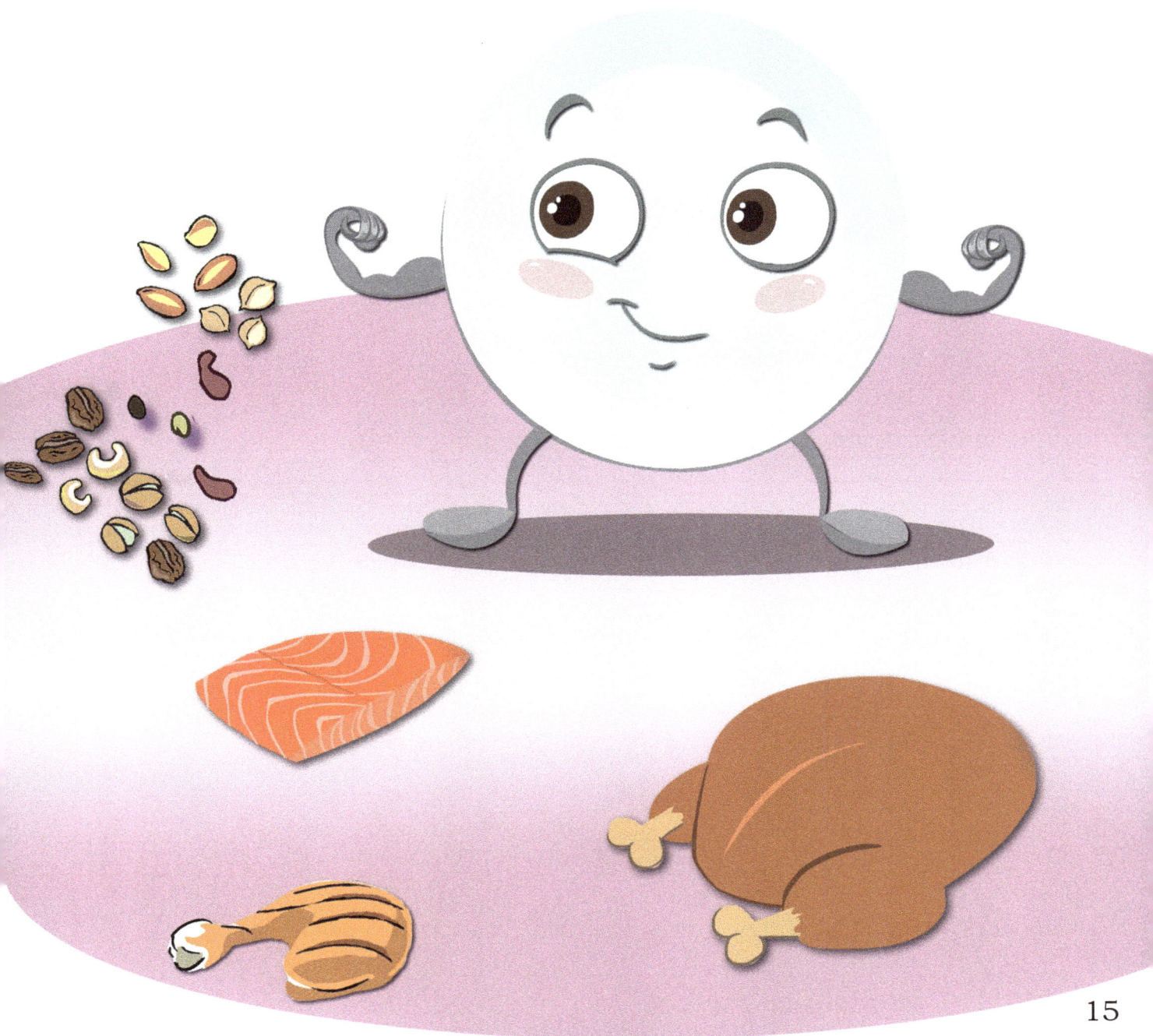

"Are you kidding?" laughed Jesse.

"No," said the plate, lifting its chin. "How do you think I keep my nice round curves?"

Then, to Jesse's disbelief, the plate began to do cartwheels and spin on its back.

"You see?" asked the plate. "Check out *those* moves!"

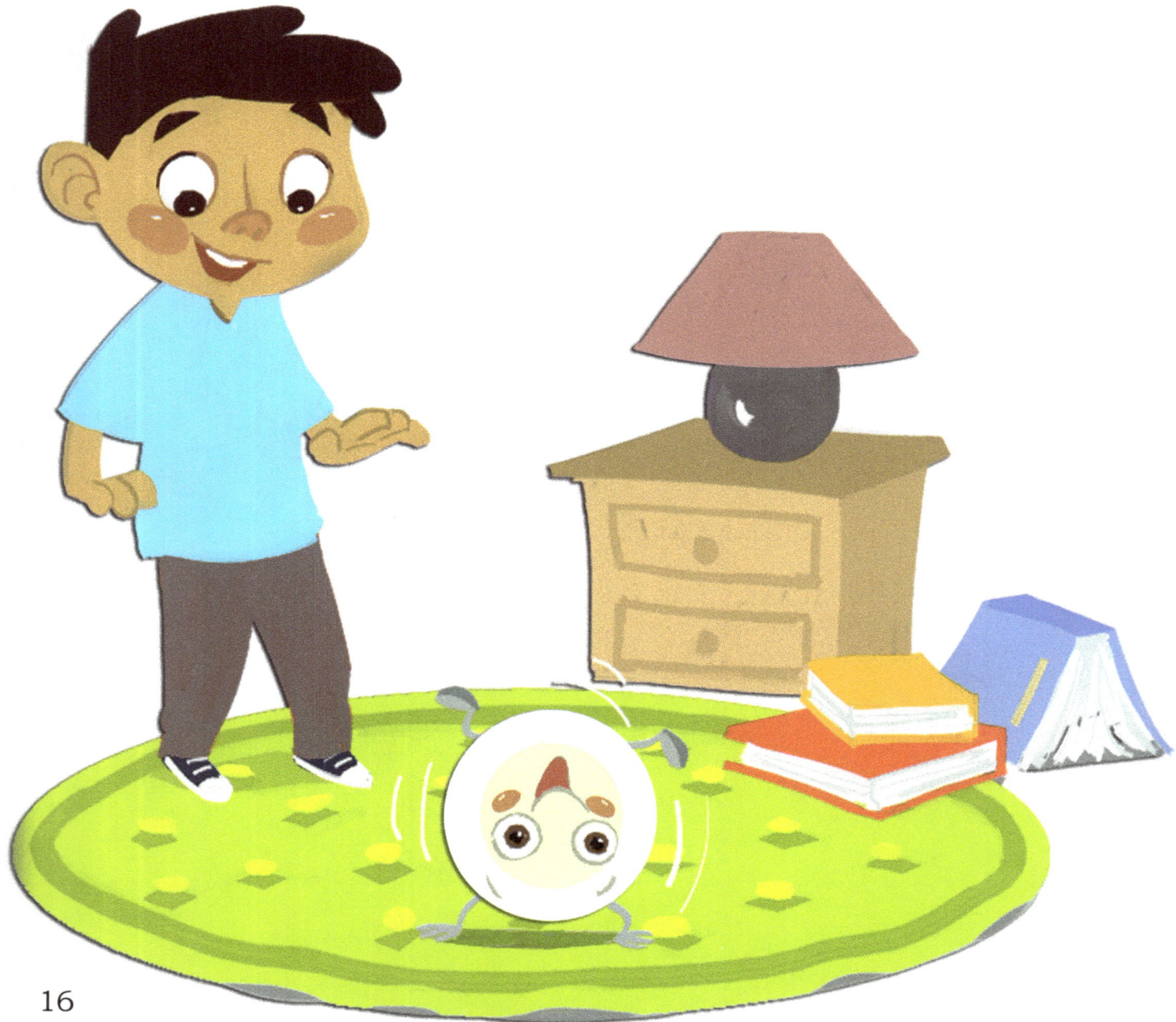

Jesse laughed with delight, blinking hard to make sure he wasn't imagining things.

When the plate stood back up, it looked a little tired.

"If you feed me even more power foods, I'll be able to play longer," it told Jesse. "Each kind of power food has its own special powers."

"What other kinds do you need?" asked Jesse.

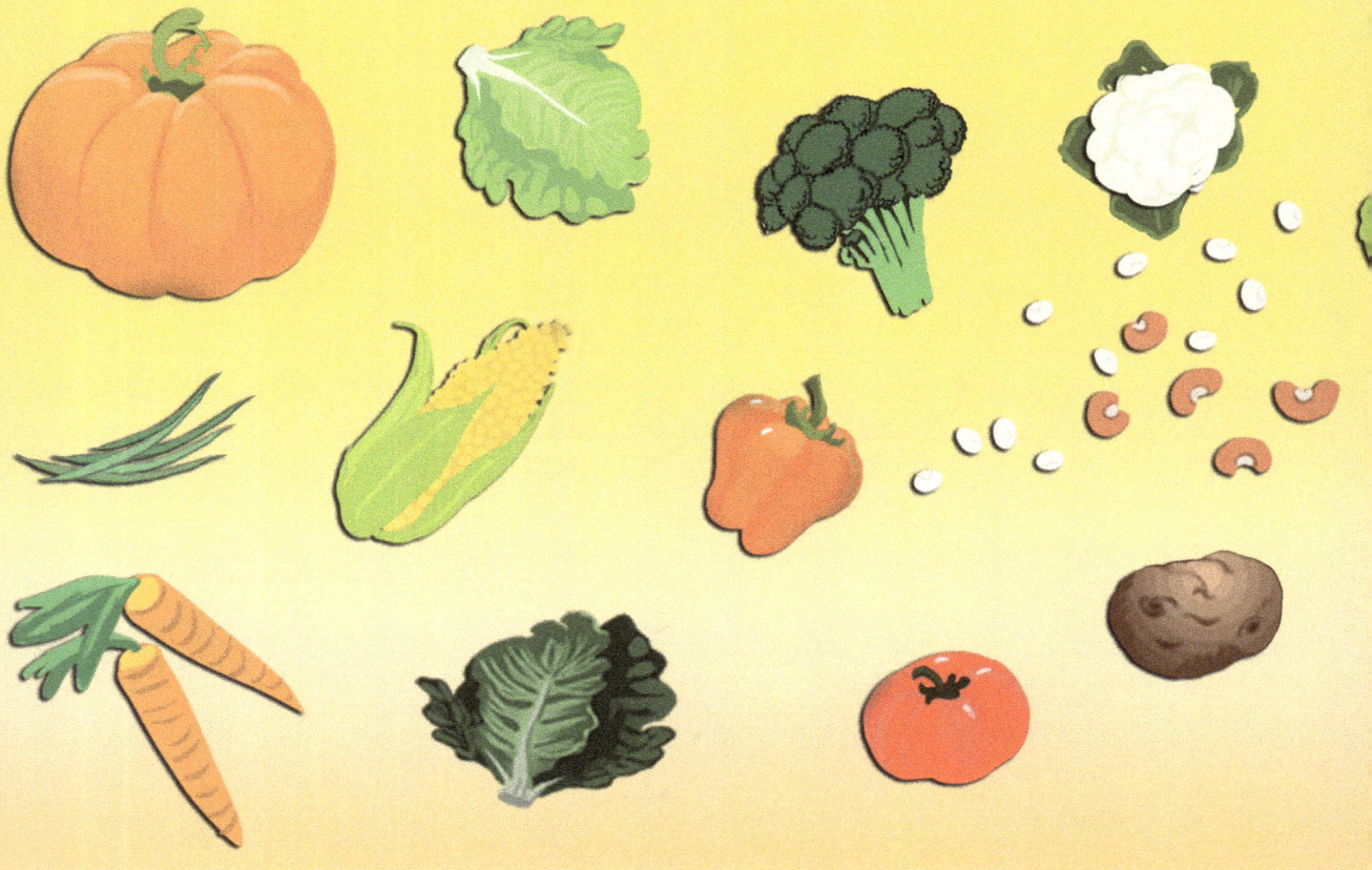

"Fruits and vegetables are two other kinds of power foods," said the plate. "*They* have the most special powers of all—especially the *colorful* ones!"

"Why is that?" asked Jesse.

"They say it's their colors that give them their special powers," said the plate, "and those special powers help keep our eyes, skin, and hearts healthy."

"Did you notice your mom eating carrots and strawberries at dinner?" asked the plate.

"Yes," said Jesse.

"She must know about super-natural power foods," said the

(For more information about Fruits and Vegetables, turn to page 86)

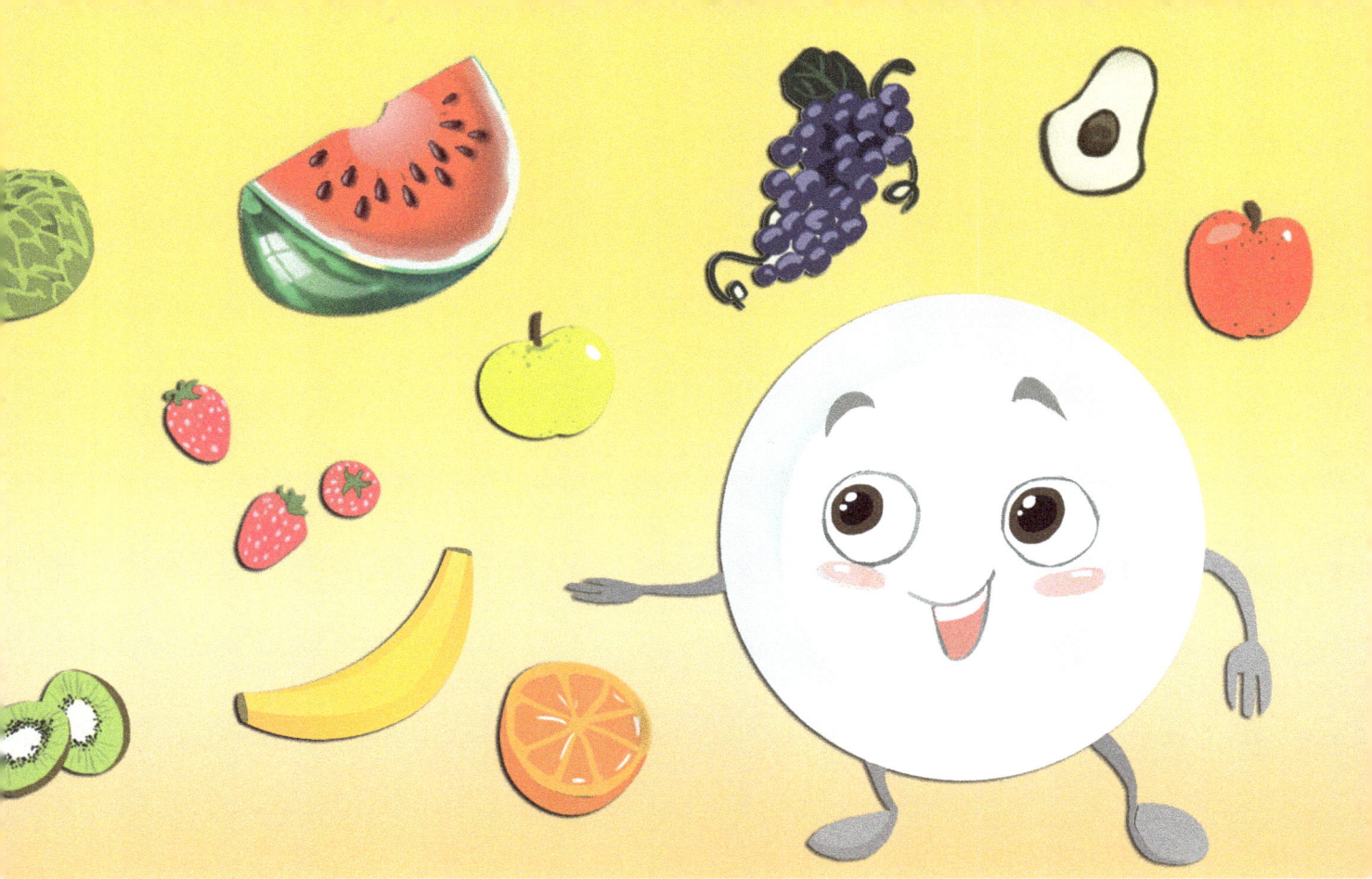

plate. "Carrots are bright orange and strawberries are bright red. They have super-natural powers!"

"Why don't grown-ups tell kids about super-natural power foods?" asked Jesse.

"Grown-ups try to tell kids all the time," said the plate, "but most kids aren't interested."

"I'm interested," said Jesse.

"Then why did you say 'no' to the carrots and strawberries?" asked the plate.

"Because," said Jesse, "I don't like carrots, and I like ice cream better than strawberries."

"Do you see what I mean?" the plate asked Jesse.

"But Mom didn't tell me that they have super-natural powers!" Jesse said.

"How many times have you heard a grown-up say, 'Eat your vegetables, they're good for you?'" asked the plate.

"Lots of times," said Jesse.

"Did you do it?" asked the plate.

"No," said Jesse. "Who believes that?"

"Would you have believed your mom if she told you they have super-natural powers?" the plate asked.

"Maybe not," said Jesse.

"Did you like riding your bicycle the first few times you tried?" the plate asked.

"No," said Jesse, "it was really hard."

"Aren't you glad you kept trying?" asked the plate.

"Of course," said Jesse, "I love riding my bicycle now."

"It's the same with super-natural power foods," said the plate. "We enjoy feeling our best when we eat them, but it may take practice to like some of them."

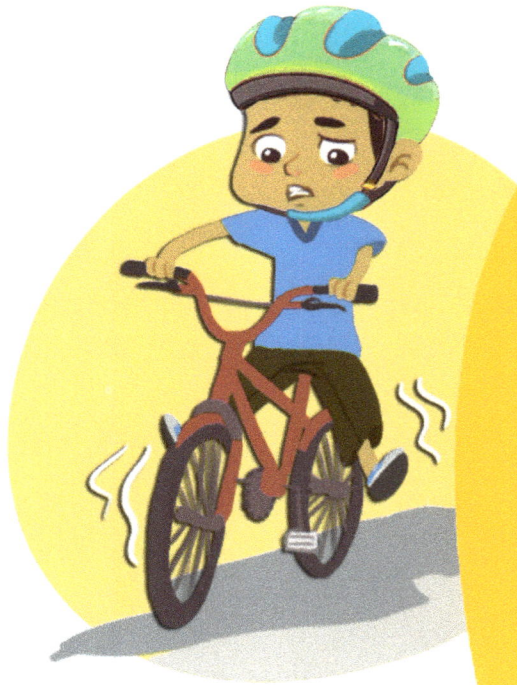
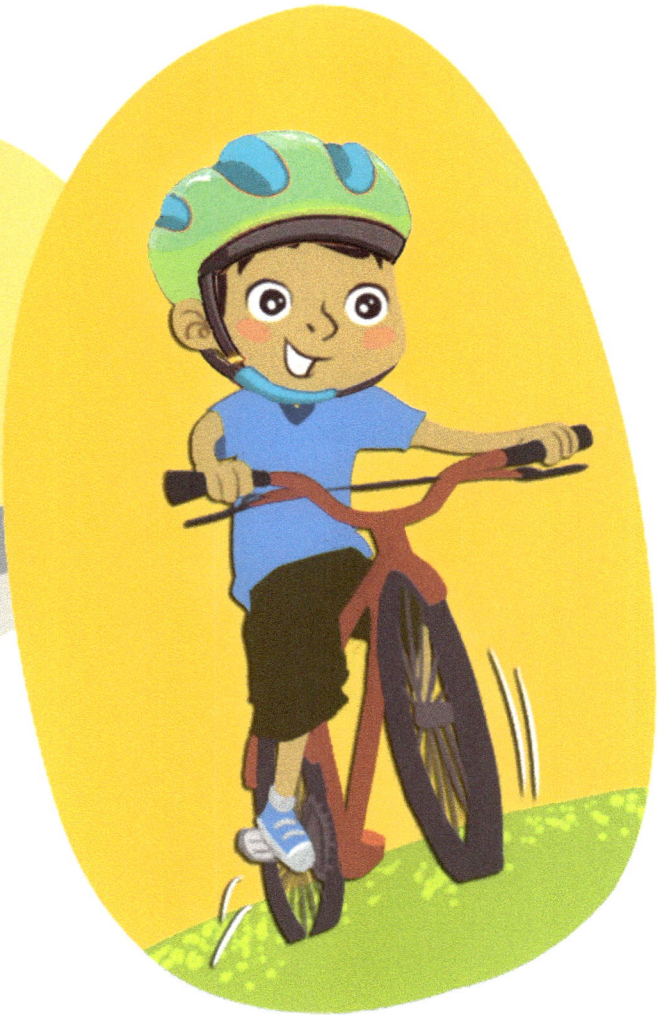

"Do you think I can learn to like vegetables just by practicing?" asked Jesse.

"Sure," said the plate, "but there may be lots of colorful fruits and vegetables that you already like."

Jesse thought about that.

"Sweet potatoes?" he asked.

"Yes!" said the plate.

"Peaches?" asked Jesse.

"Excellent!" the plate said.

"Cantaloupe, green beans, tomatoes, oranges, watermelon, grapes. . .," Jesse went on and on.

"Fabulous!" cheered the plate. "You've got the picture!"

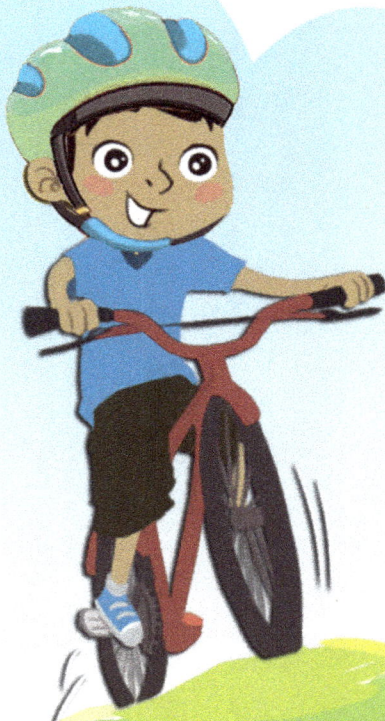

4

RED AND GREEN

The next night at dinner, Jesse's mom served beans, brown rice, green spinach salad, and red watermelon.

Jesse said "yes" to beans and rice, and also to spinach salad. He didn't really *want* to eat spinach, but he wanted to help his plate.

Slowly, Jesse began to taste the spinach. To his surprise, it didn't taste so bad. He tried some more and managed to eat a few bites, all the while thinking about how wonderful he felt when riding his bicycle.

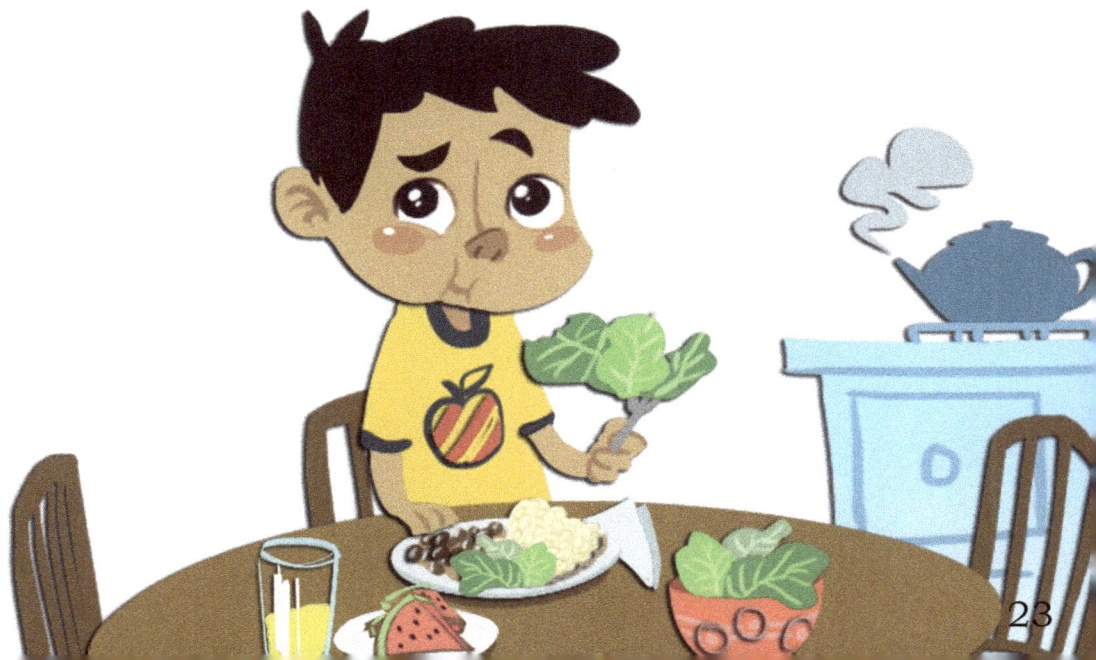

For dessert, Jesse was happy to eat red watermelon. It was one of his favorite foods.

Next, Jesse's mom offered him cookies, but he felt too full to eat them.

After dinner, back in Jesse's room, the plate was smiling from rim to rim.

"Jesse, you're the best! I haven't felt this wonderful since my last home," it said, giving Jesse a big hug.

Jesse felt great, too. He had an easy time doing his homework that night. The plate could even read well enough to help Jesse study for his spelling test.

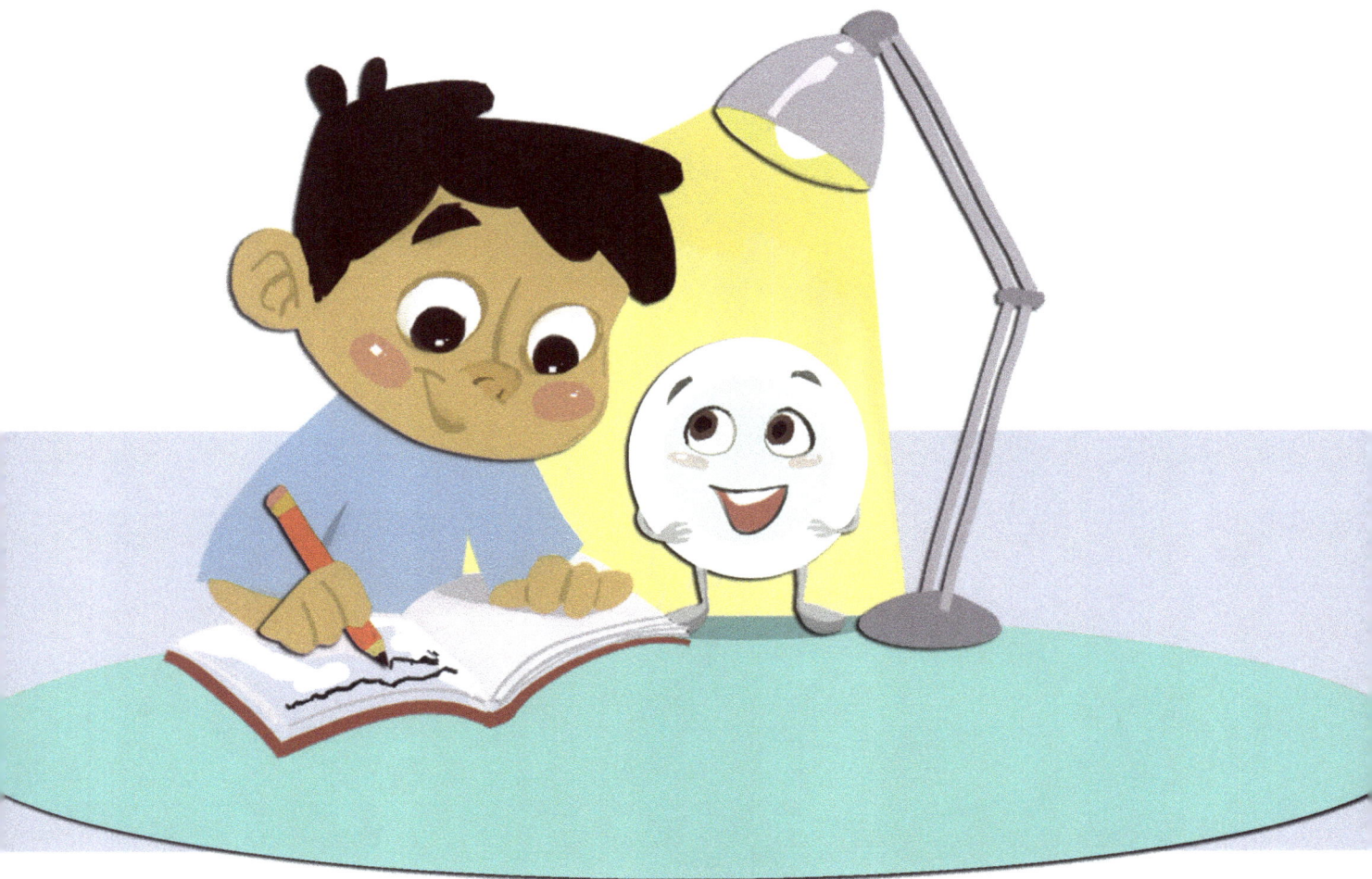

When the plate finished helping Jesse with his homework, it began to brush itself off.

"What are you doing?" laughed Jesse.

"I'm brushing off the extra salt I got today," the plate said. "Too much salt isn't healthy for us."

"How did you get too much salt?" asked Jesse. "I didn't add salt to my food today."

"That's true," said the plate, "but salt often gets added to foods in other ways. I can teach you how to watch out for that."

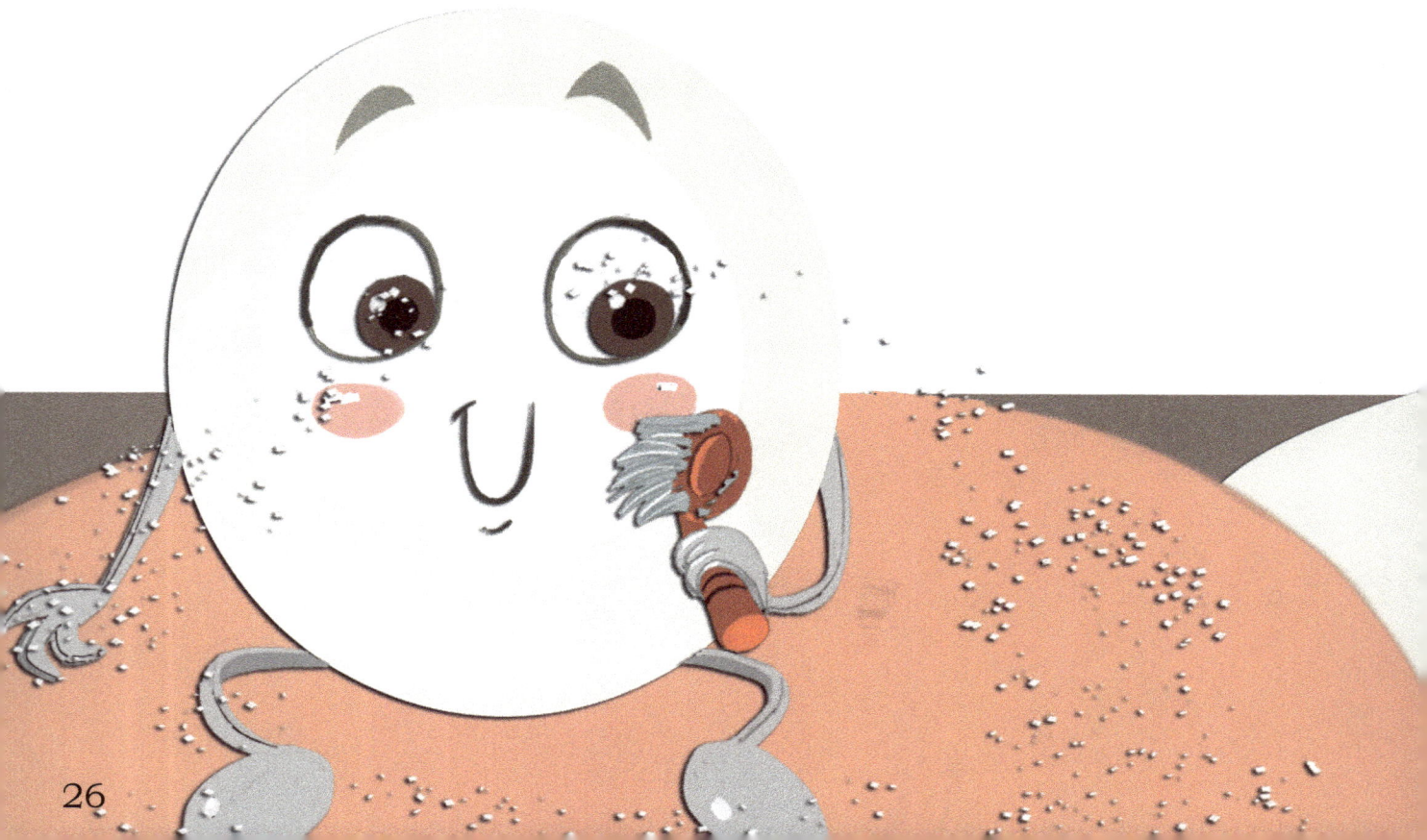

5

PLATE TRICKS

A few days later, the plate worked up the courage to ask, "Jesse, may I please go to school with you one day?"

"I'm not sure," said Jesse. "What if you break in my backpack?"

"If you help me get even stronger, I'm sure I'll be okay," said the plate. "All the kids used to take me to school with them. How do you think I learned how to read?"

"How strong are you now?" Jesse asked.

"Pretty strong," said the plate, trying to flex a muscle, "but there's another kind of super-natural power food that I need . . ."

"Here we go again," said Jesse. "What now?"

"Dairy foods," said the plate. "Have you noticed that your mom drinks low-fat milk, and eats foods made from milk, like cheese and yogurt? Those are dairy foods. Foods made with milk have super-natural powers that keep our bones and teeth strong."

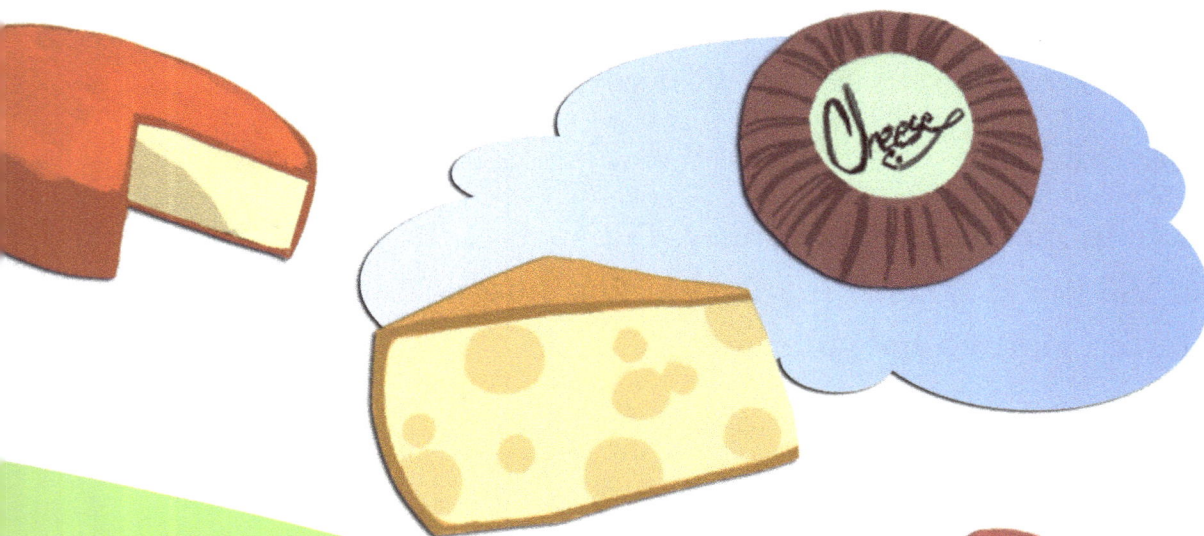

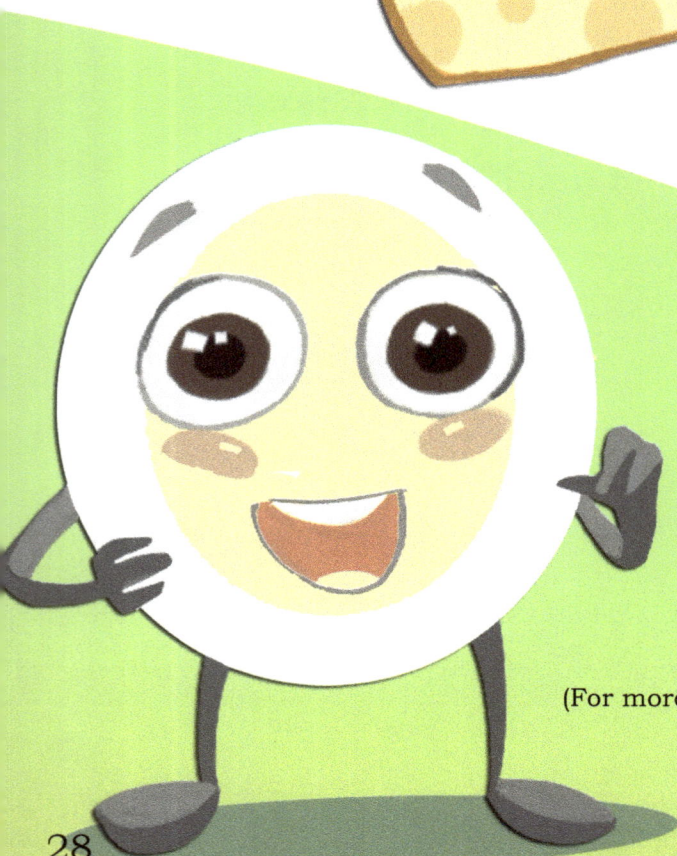

(For more information about Dairy Foods, turn to page 90)

"But you're flat," said Jesse. "You can't hold milk, or even cereal with milk."

"Well," said the plate as it stuck out its chest and stood up taller, "you know how you've been feeding me so many power foods, Jesse?"

"Yes," said Jesse.

"Guess what?" asked the plate. "I've been practicing really hard, and I have a surprise for you!"

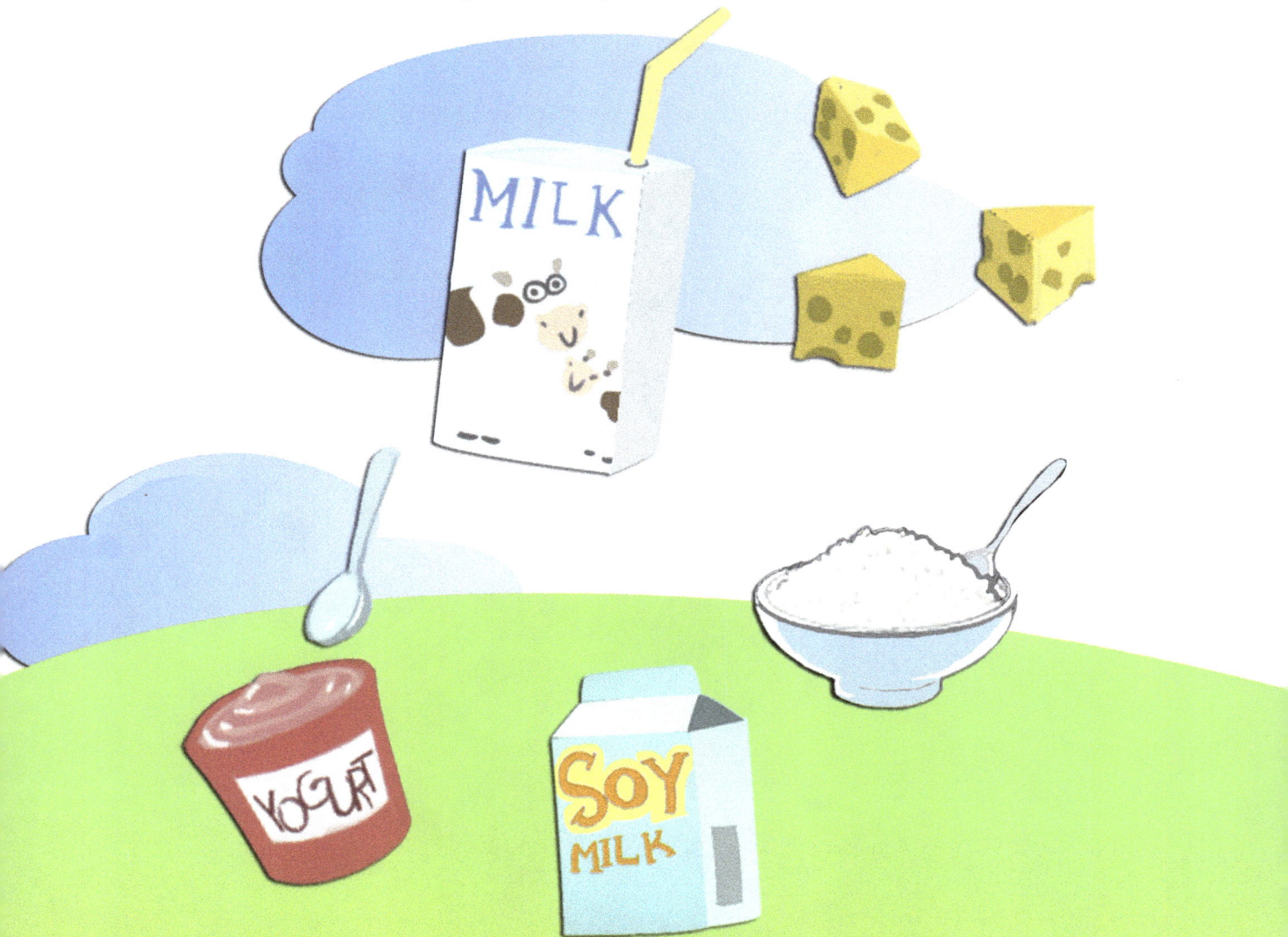

"You do?" asked Jesse. He loved surprises.

"Yes!" said the plate. "Because of your help, I'm getting better every day!"

"I can't believe you're still trying to be better than just a plate," said Jesse.

"You bet I am!" said the plate. "I never give up. Watch this!"

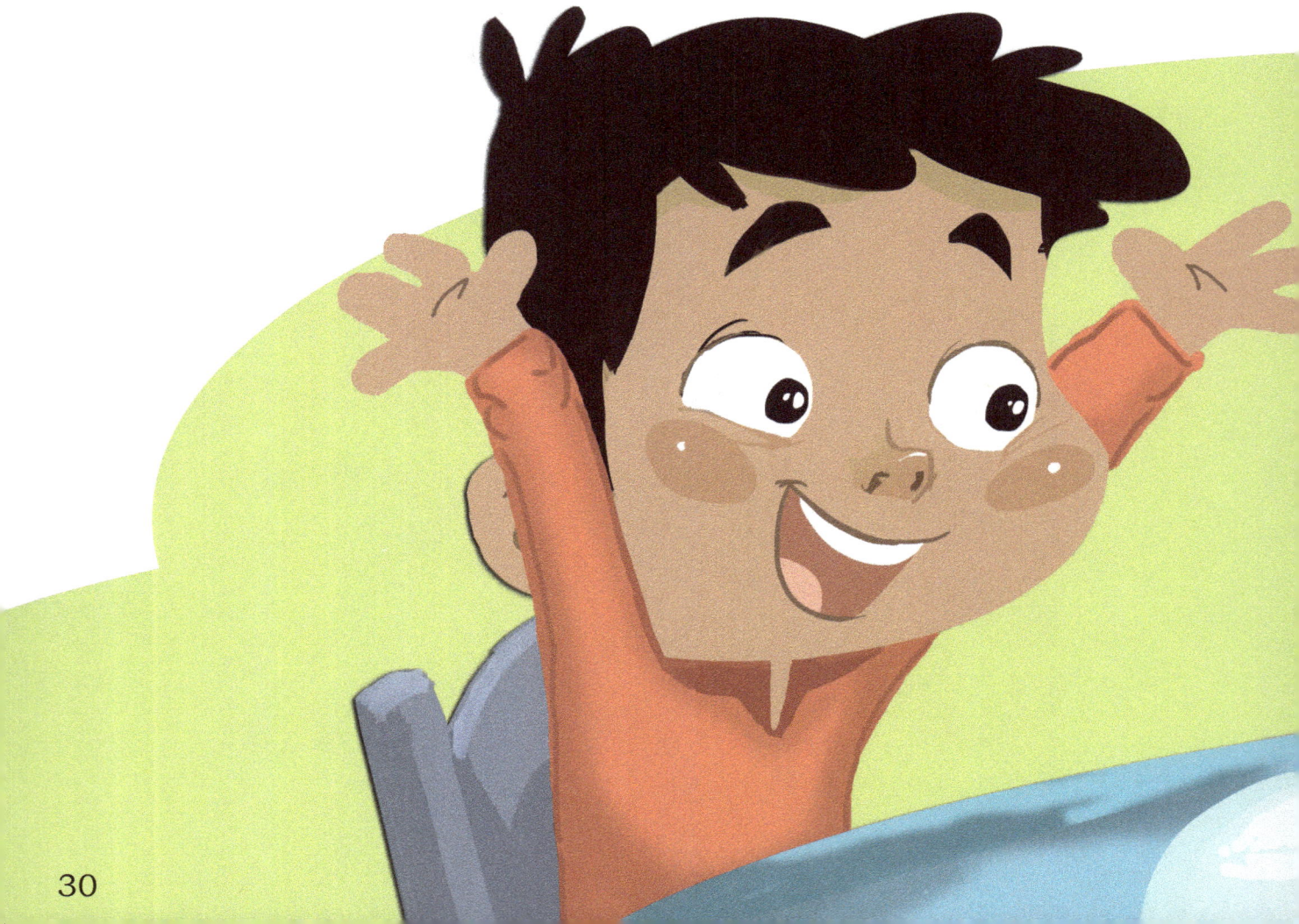

As Jesse watched, the plate took a deep breath and began to rock, swivel, tilt, and turn. Then, sure enough, its edges began to curl up. Little by little, its sides lifted, until the plate, straining with effort, turned into a bowl!

"WOW!" yelled Jesse. "That's the best trick I've ever seen!"

"You see?" beamed the plate. "I *can* be better than just a plate! I can be a plate *or* a bowl!"

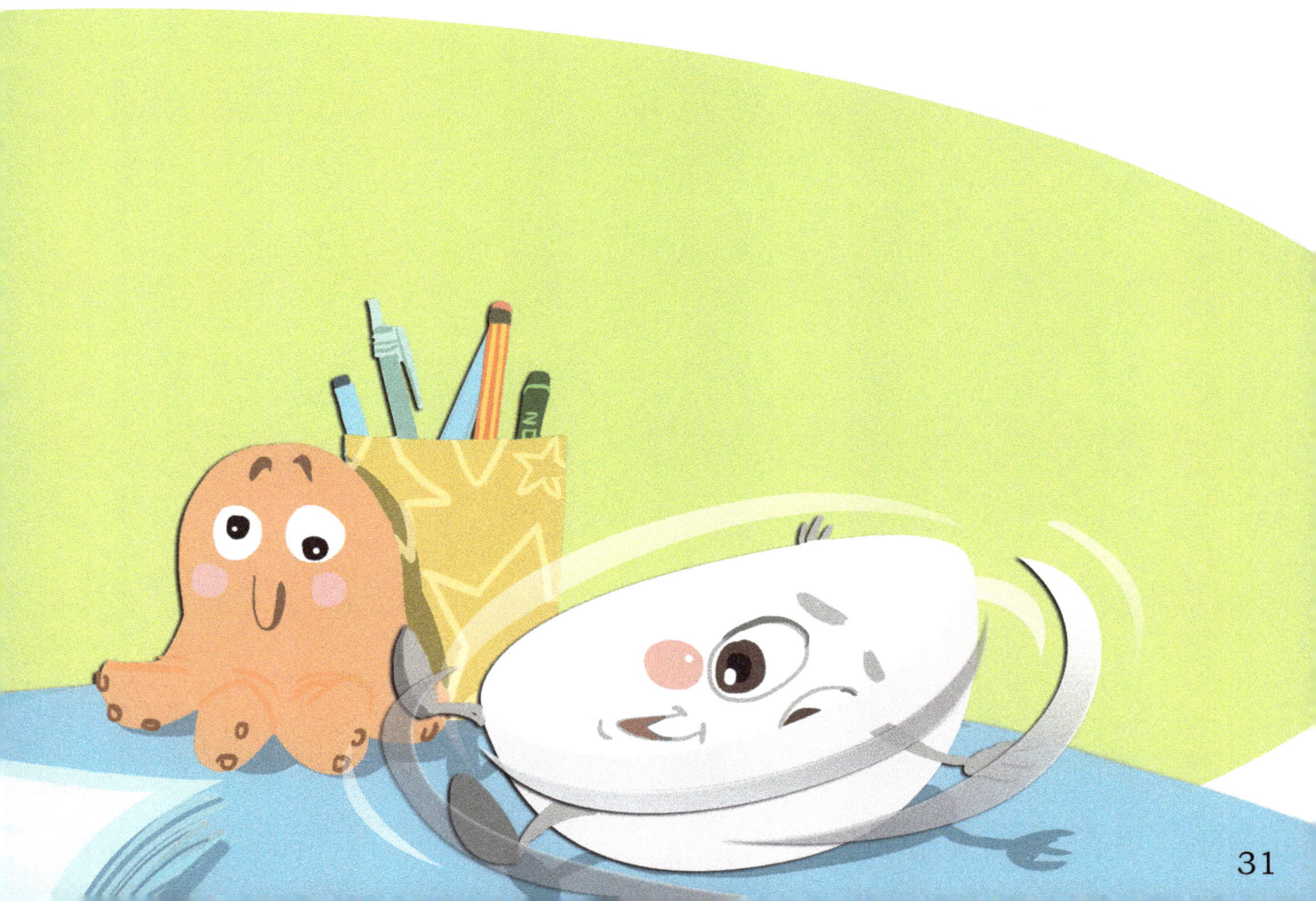

"How long can you stay like that?" Jesse asked the plate.

"Well," said the plate, trying hard to hold up its sides, "if you keep feeding me dairy foods to keep my bones strong, and energy foods like whole grain breads and cereals, I can keep my sides up even longer."

"Whole grain *what*?" asked Jesse.

"Whole grains," said the plate. "You've never heard of whole grains? Whole wheat bread, brown rice, oatmeal . . ."

"I didn't know those were whole *anything*," said Jesse.

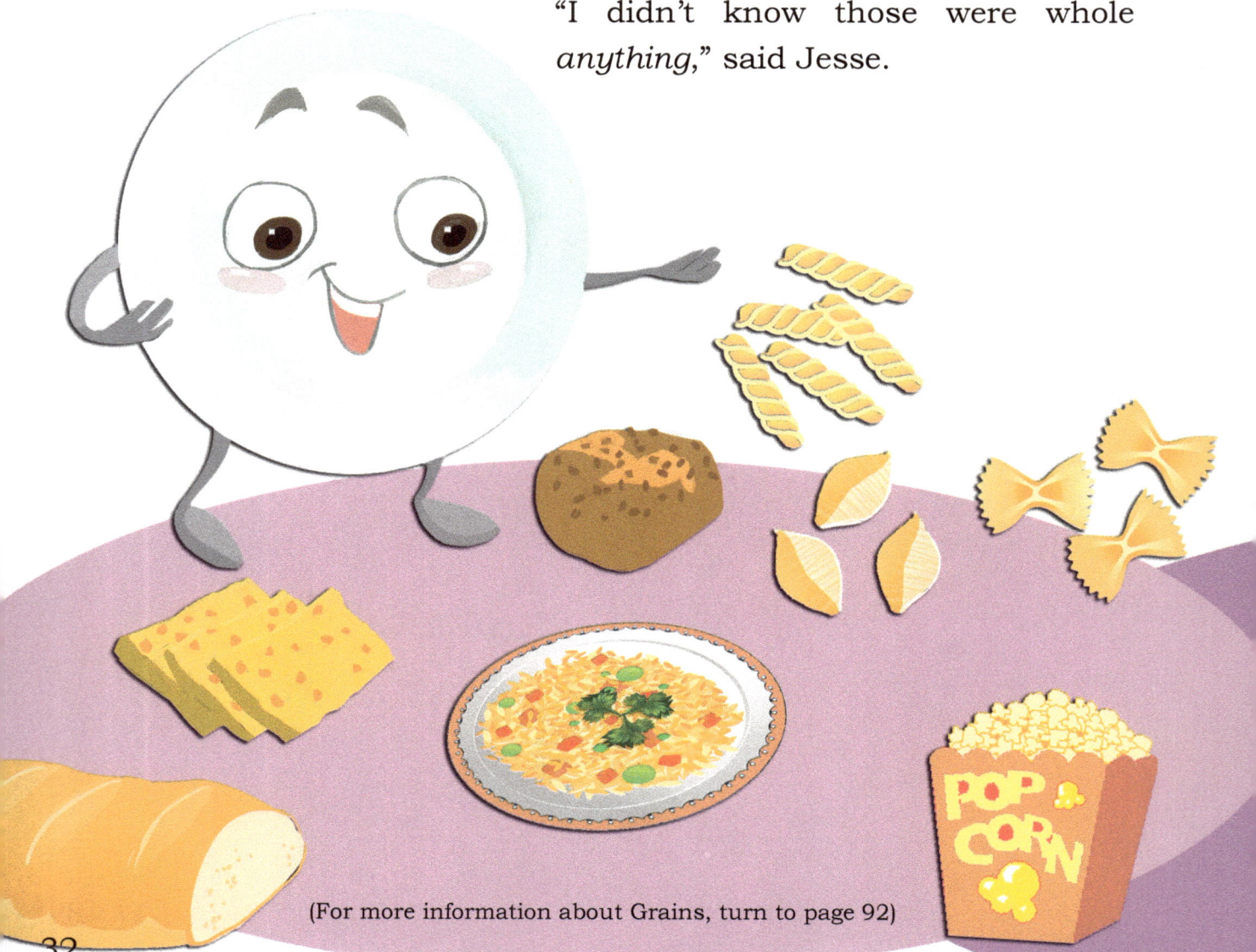

(For more information about Grains, turn to page 92)

"Uh-oh," said the plate. "Well, never mind. Your mom's on it. I saw her serve whole wheat pasta the other night. I'll teach you more about that later on."

"Anyway," the plate continued, "it would be a big help if you would use me for your cereal and milk. But please, if you have to add sugar, use as little as possible. Added sugar has no special powers, and too much can make us feel tired."

"Okay," said Jesse, "but how many kinds of super-natural power foods are there?"

"We need to eat foods from five different groups," said the plate, "because each group has its own special powers. The five groups are Fruits, Vegetables, Grains, Protein Foods, and Dairy."

"How can I remember all that?" asked Jesse.

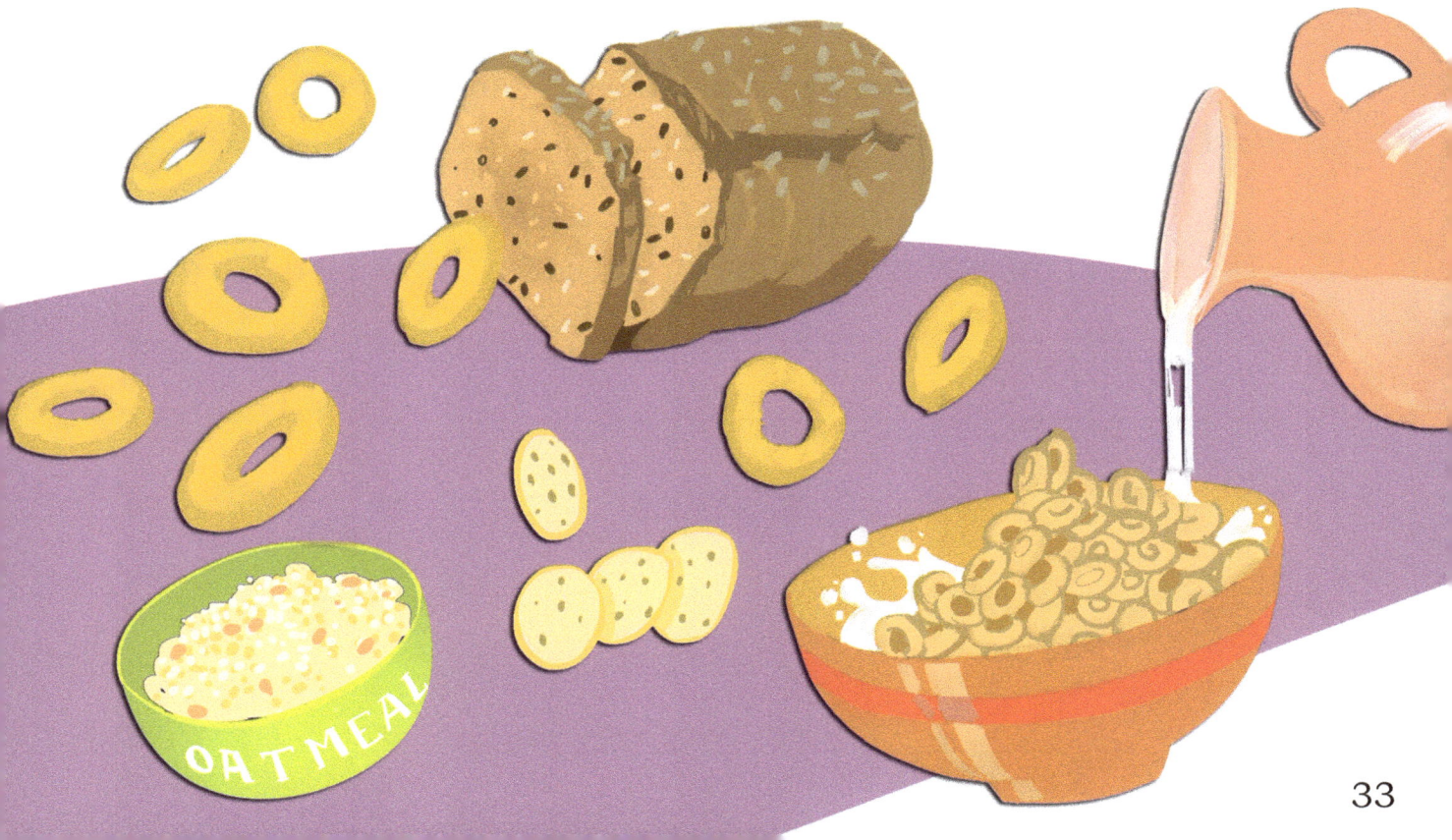

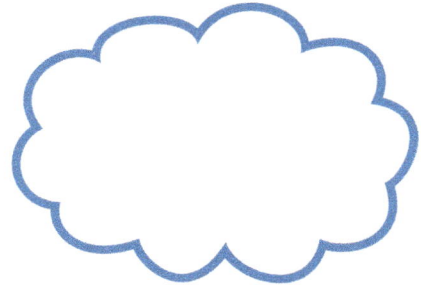

"It's easy," said the plate. "That's where Magic Plates come in. Take a look at me. How many parts do you see?"

"Five," answered Jesse. "Two arms, two legs, and...a plate?"

"That's right, Jesse," said the plate. "Now, turn me over and check me out."

Jesse turned the plate over and was amazed. The back of the plate had five sections. Each section had the name of a power food group and pictures of the power foods in that group.

Anytime Jesse turned the Magic Plate over, he would be reminded of the power foods he should eat to be the best he could be.

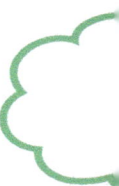

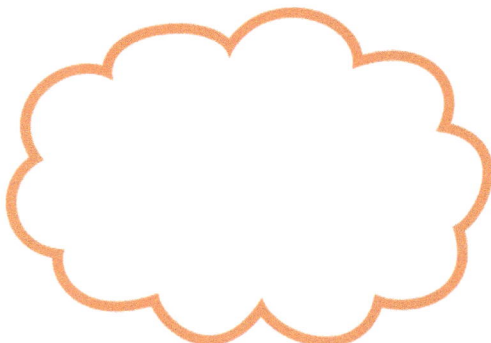

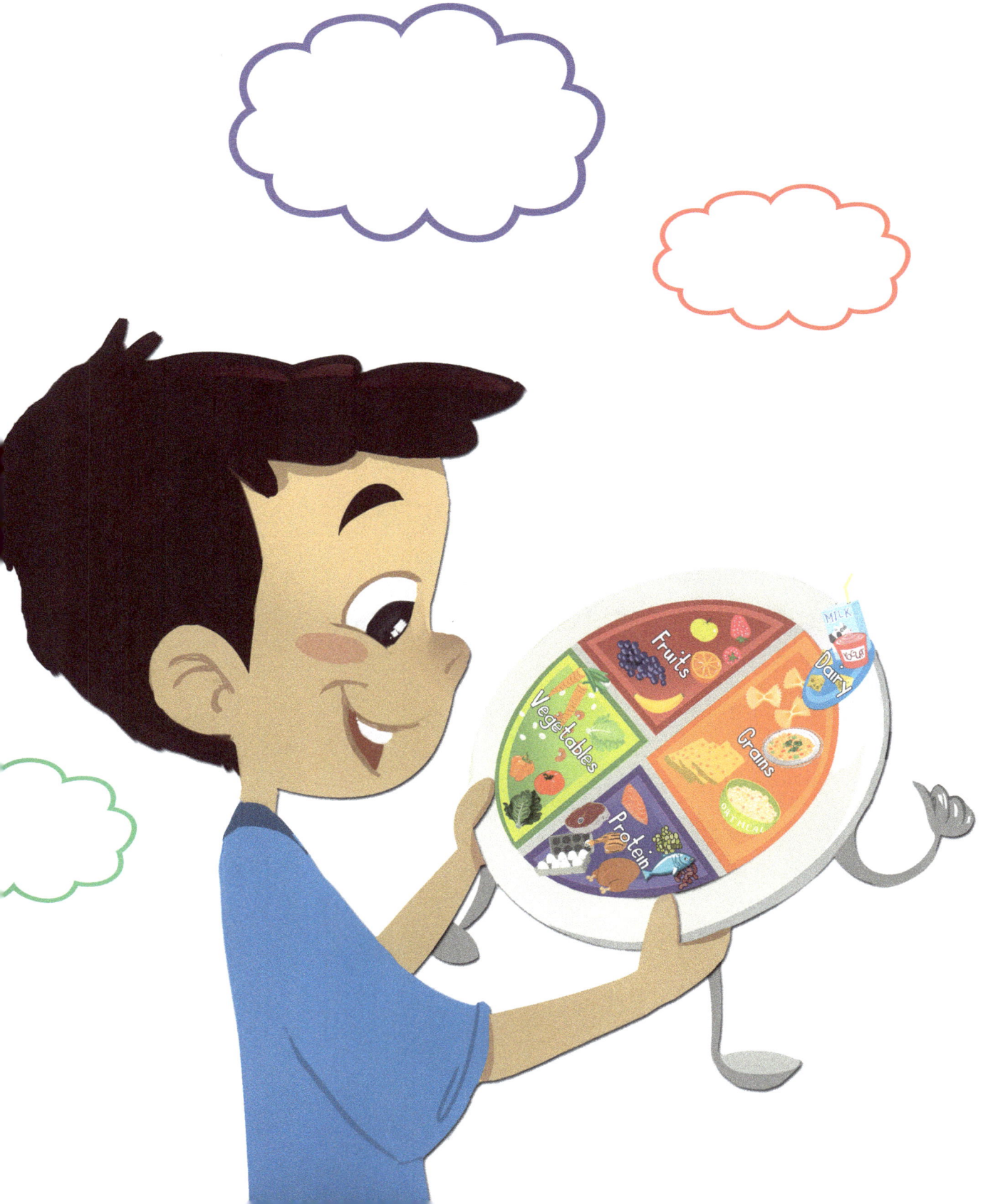

From that time on, the plate did its bowl trick each morning, and Jesse ate his whole grain cereal with milk and just a little bit of added sugar.

Jesse also ate many other super-natural power foods from his Magic Plate, and he and his plate grew healthy and strong.

To Jesse's delight, his softball team was starting to win again, and his grades were improving, too!

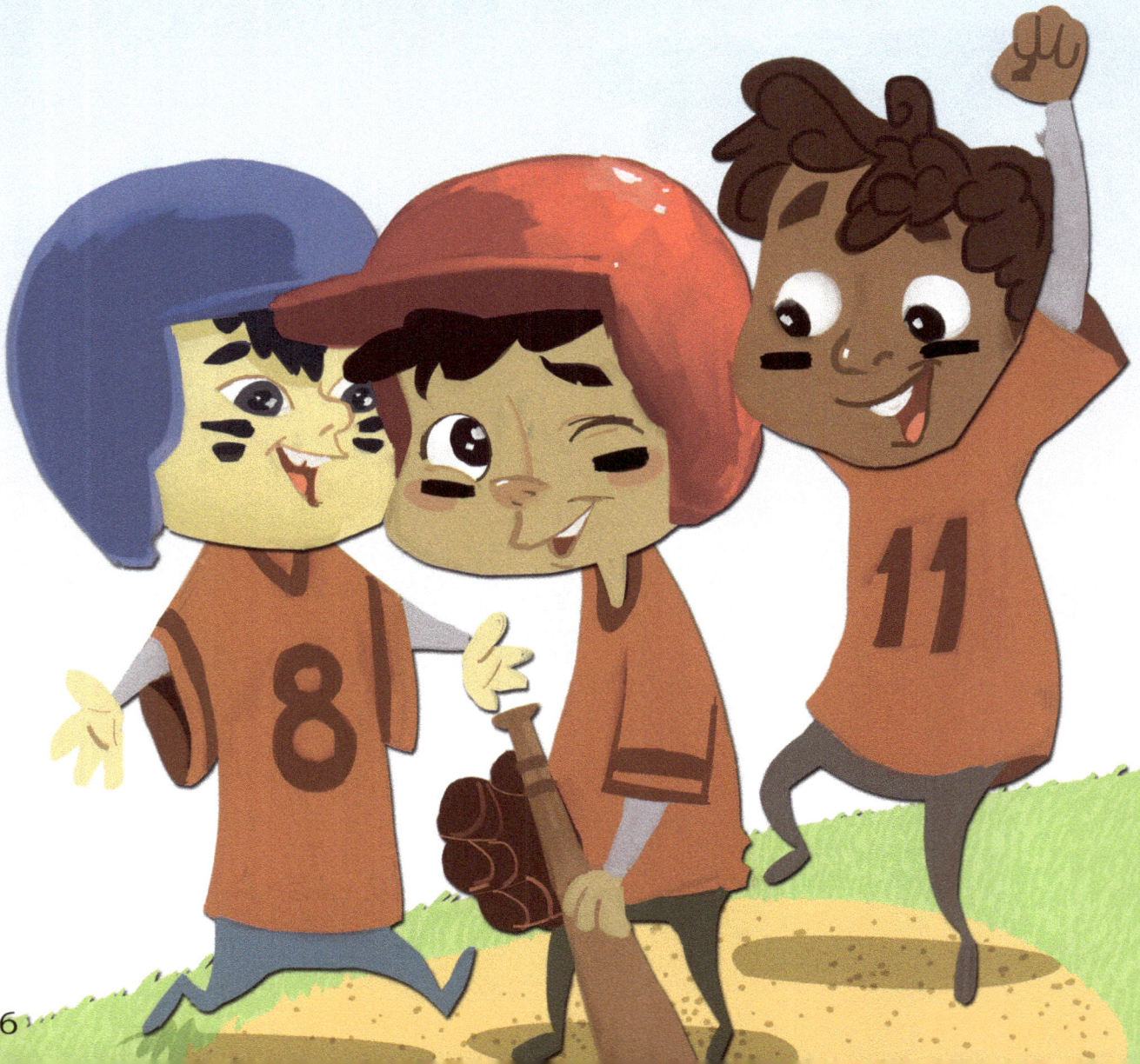

6
SHOW AND TELL

One day, Jesse's teacher announced that the class would be having 'Show and Tell' in two weeks.

Jesse was sure that his Magic Plate would be proud to be shown off. But the plate wasn't happy about it at all.

"What's the matter?" asked Jesse. "Don't you want to be my 'Show and Tell' project? I thought you'd be excited."

"I'm sorry, Jesse," said the plate, sadly. "I'd love to meet your friends, but I'm not shiny anymore. I don't want to look like a dull plate in front of your class."

"I'm proud of you just the way you are," said Jesse. "Is there anything I can do to help?"

"There may be something. I'm just not sure it will work," said the plate.

"What is it?" asked Jesse.

"I need a little bit of oil," said the plate. "Oils have special powers that help my coating. Would you be willing to try some? Please use just a *tiny little bit*, though. I don't want to get greasy."

"Okay," said Jesse. "Let's give it a try."

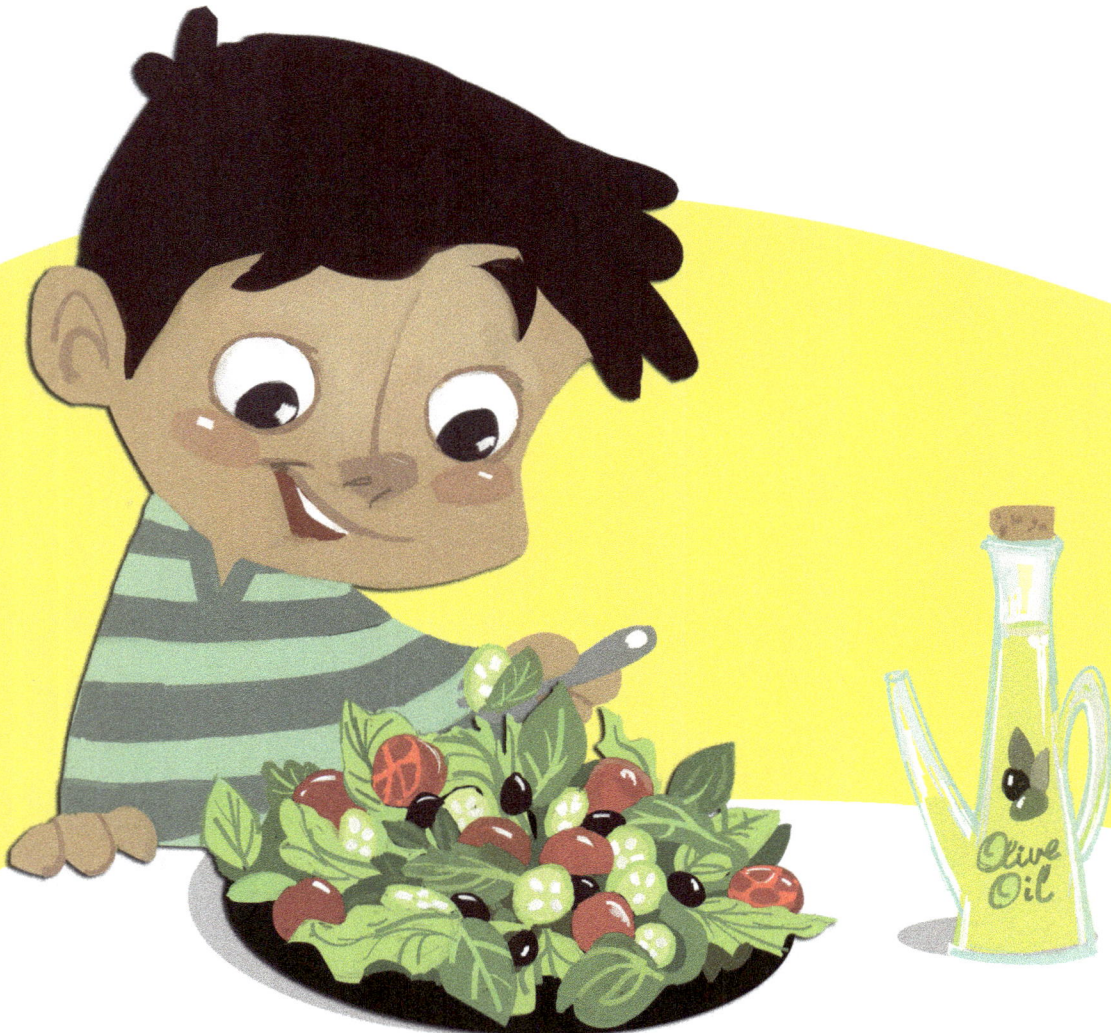

That night at dinner, Jesse enjoyed eating a salad with just a little bit of oil in the dressing.

Another day, instead of buttering his bread, Jesse poured just a little vegetable oil onto his plate and dipped his bread in it. He liked the way it tasted.

With each passing day, the plate became shinier and shinier. Jesse felt great, too!

(For more information about Oils, turn to page 94)

On the day of 'Show and Tell,' Jesse's mom helped him wrap his Magic Plate to protect it on the way to school.

When it was Jesse's turn for 'Show and Tell,' he pulled his strong, healthy, shiny plate from his backpack, unwrapped it, and walked up to the front of the class.

"This is my Magic Plate," said Jesse, holding the plate up so everyone could see it.

"What would you like to tell us about your Magic Plate, Jesse?" his teacher asked.

"My Magic Plate teaches me really cool things," said Jesse. "I've learned how important it is to take good care of our plates, so they can be their best. When our plates are the best they can be, they help us become the best that we can be."

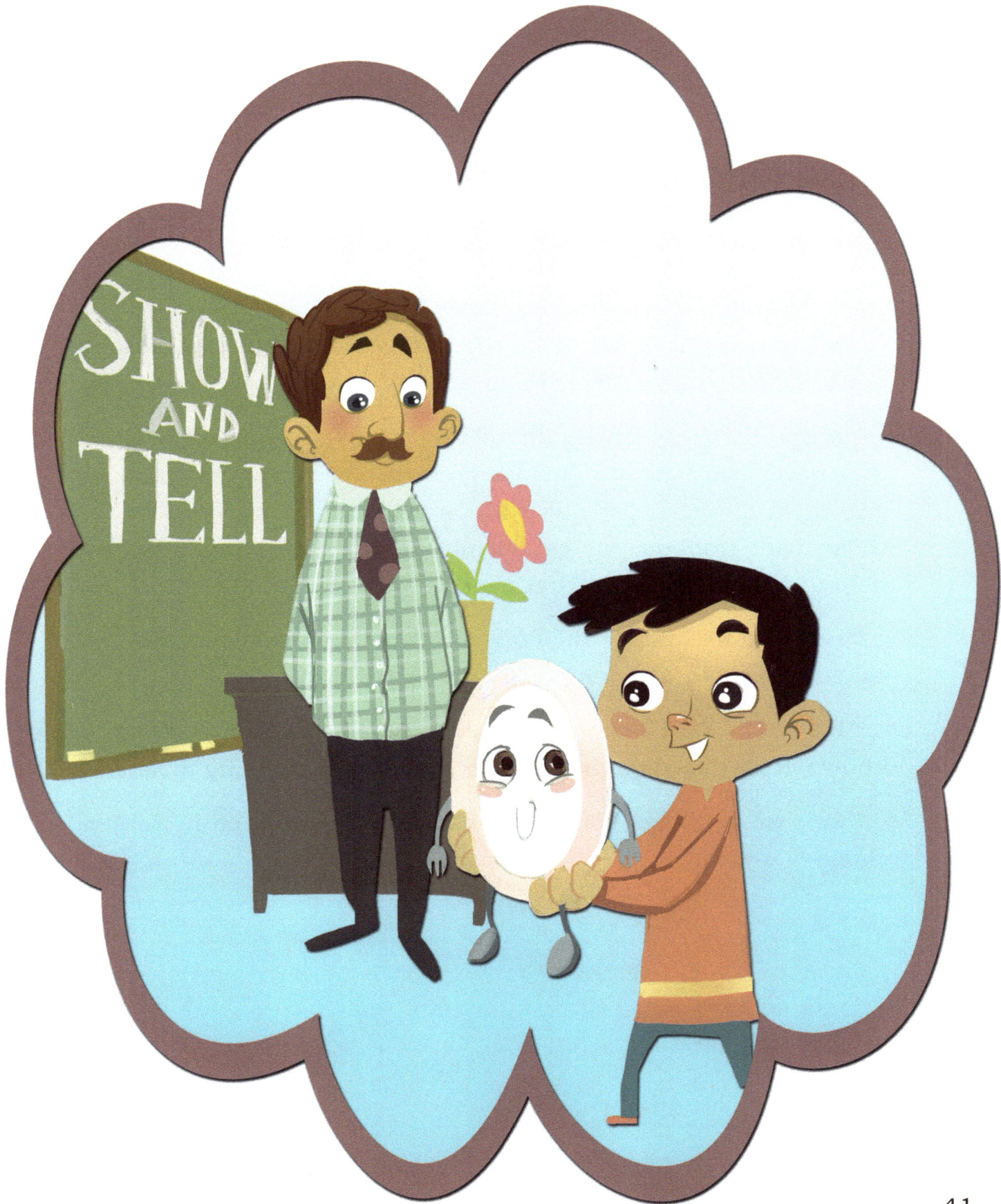

"It's wonderful to try to be the best we can be," said Jesse's teacher. "How can a Magic Plate help us do that?"

"Magic Plates teach us about the super-natural power foods they need," said Jesse. "We take good care of our plates when we give them lots of super-natural power foods. Then, when we eat those foods from our plates, our plates take good care of *us*, and help *us* become the best that *we* can be."

"How can we know what foods are super-natural power foods?" asked Jesse's teacher.

"It's easy," said Jesse. "A Magic Plate will share everything it knows. It just needs to belong to someone who's willing to listen."

"Can we get Magic Plates, too?" asked the children in Jesse's class.

"Sure you can," answered Jesse. "Magic Plates can be anywhere."

"But the *best* magic," Jesse continued, "is in the *special powers* that nature gives its foods, to keep us healthy and strong."

"One more thing," Jesse added. "Never turn down a shopping trip with your mom!"

Then, to the delight of everyone, the plate looked right at Jesse's classmates, smiled broadly, and winked.

THE END

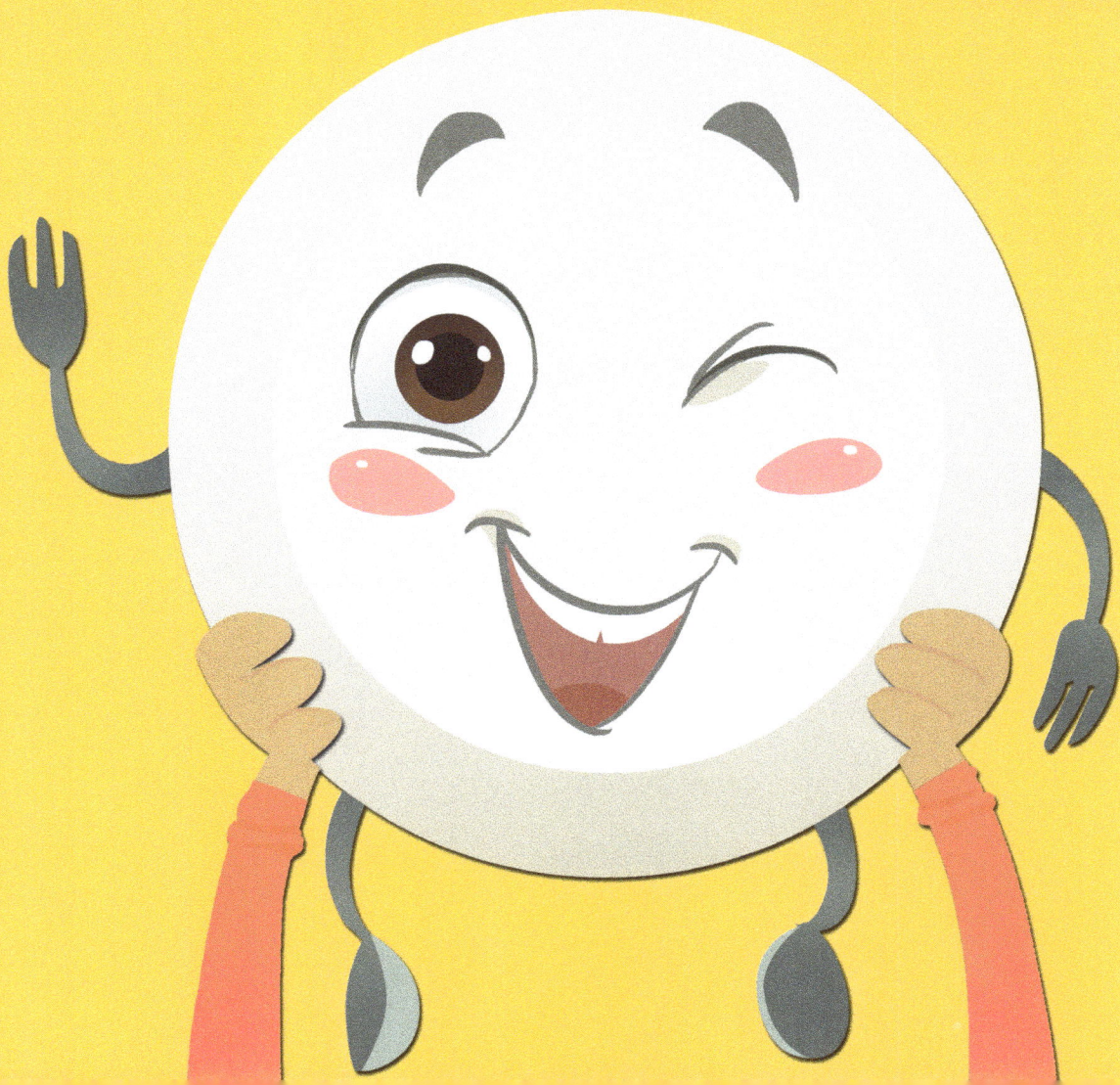

PART TWO

HOW TO MAKE YOUR OWN MAGIC PLATE

SUPPLIES NEEDED:

1 Paper plate (9 inch size works best)

Scissors

Stick glue

Clear tape

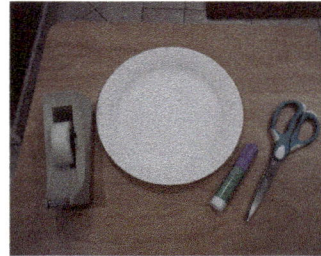

DIRECTIONS

1. Ask a grown-up to help you cut out circles A and B (see pages 49-53).

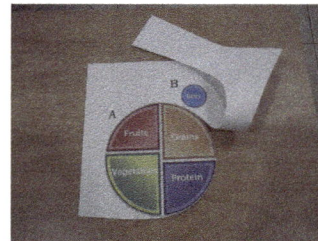

2. Glue both circles to the back of your paper plate.

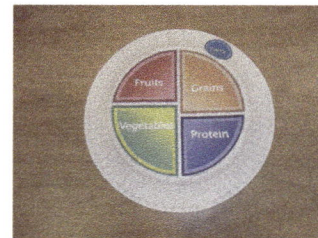

3. Choose a Magic Plate face (see pages 55-63), and ask a grown-up to help you cut it out.

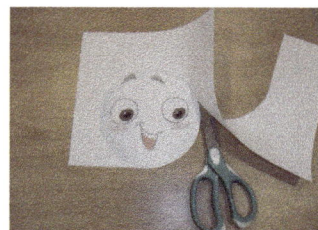

4. Glue the face to the front of the plate.

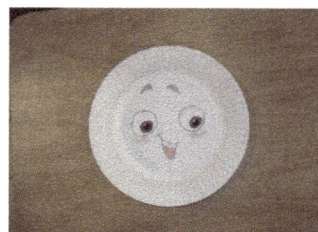

(continued)

5. Select your Magic Plate left and right arms (see pages 65-71), and ask a grown-up to help you cut them out.

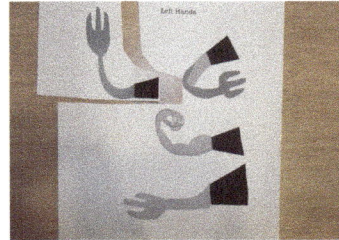

6. Tape the arms to the back of the plate, with the white side of the arms facing you.

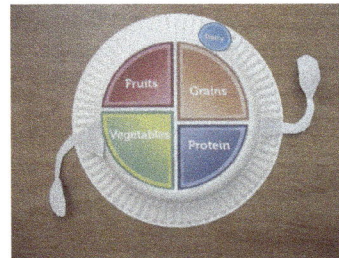

7. Select your Magic Plate legs (see pages 73-75), and ask a grown-up to help you cut them out.

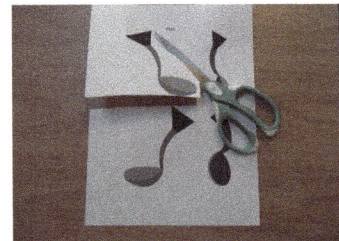

8. Tape the legs to the back of the plate, with the white side of the legs facing you.

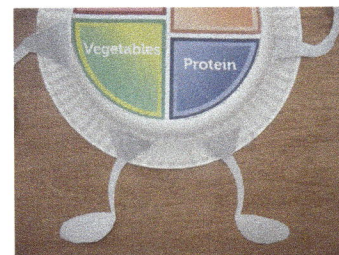

(continued)

9. Ask a grown-up to help you cut out the pictures of the food groups (see pages 77-81).

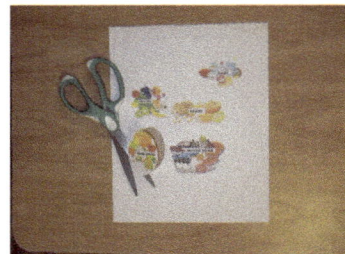

10. Glue each food group within its correct section on the back of the plate.

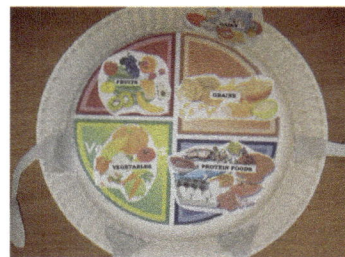

11. Now you have a Magic Plate!

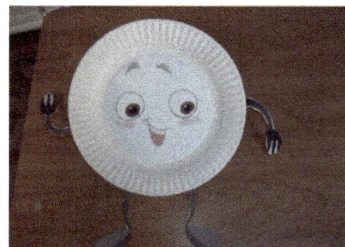

A

B

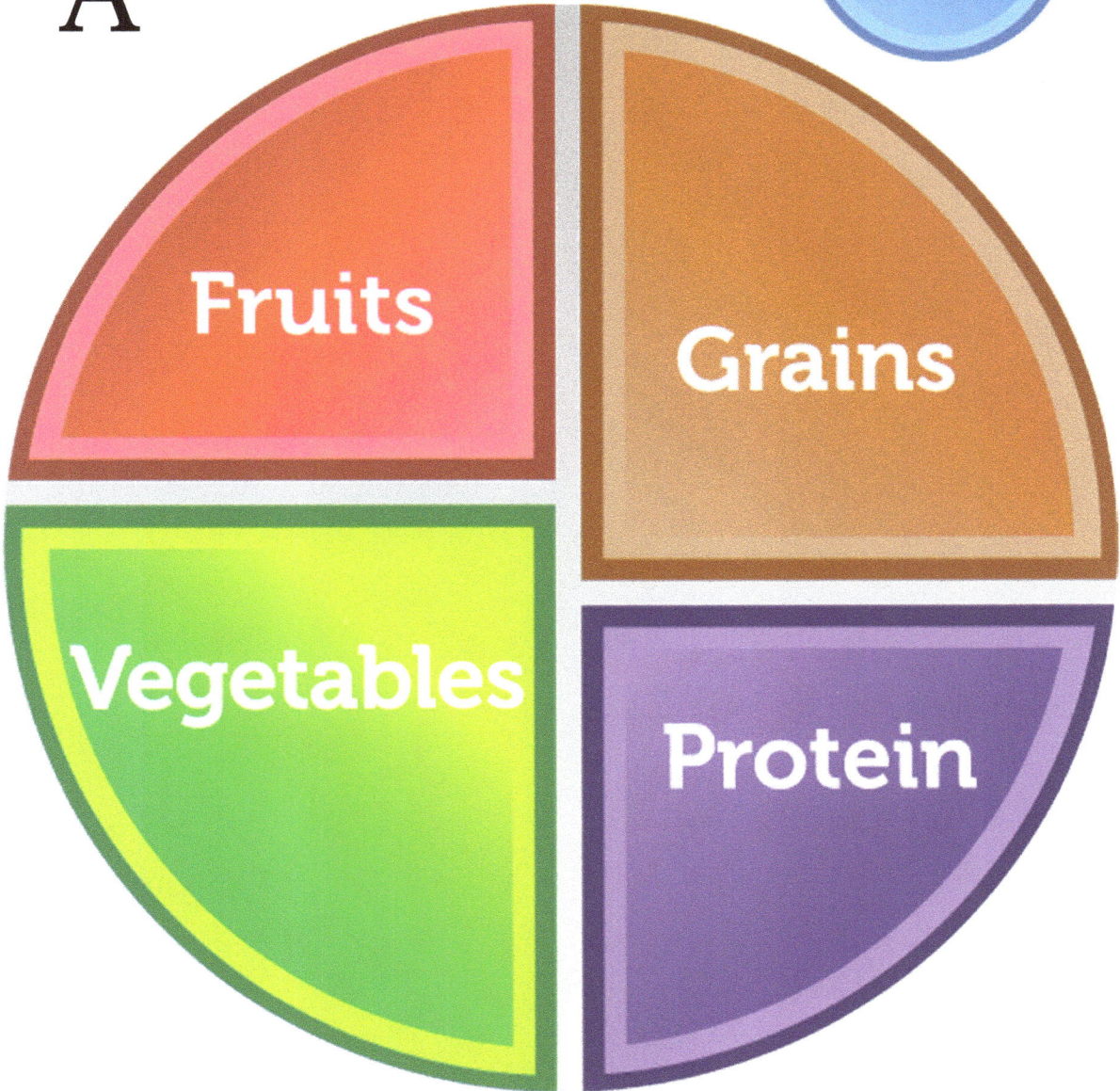

Dairy

Fruits

Grains

Vegetables

Protein

B

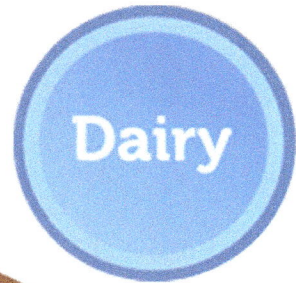

Dairy

A

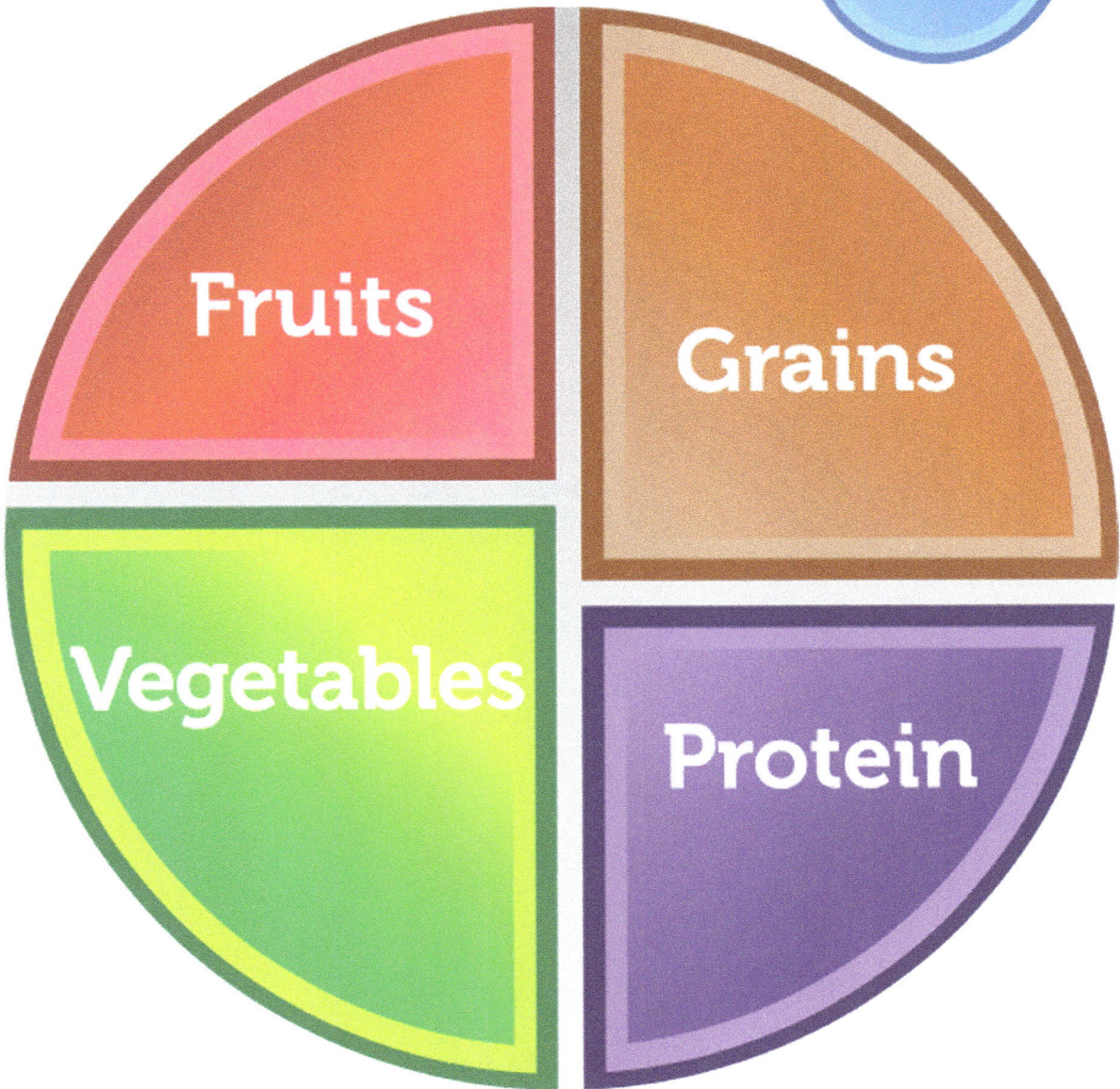

Fruits

Grains

Vegetables

Protein

B

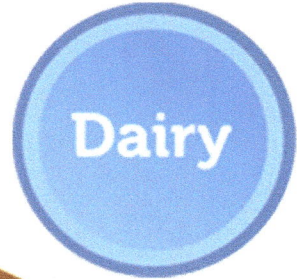

A

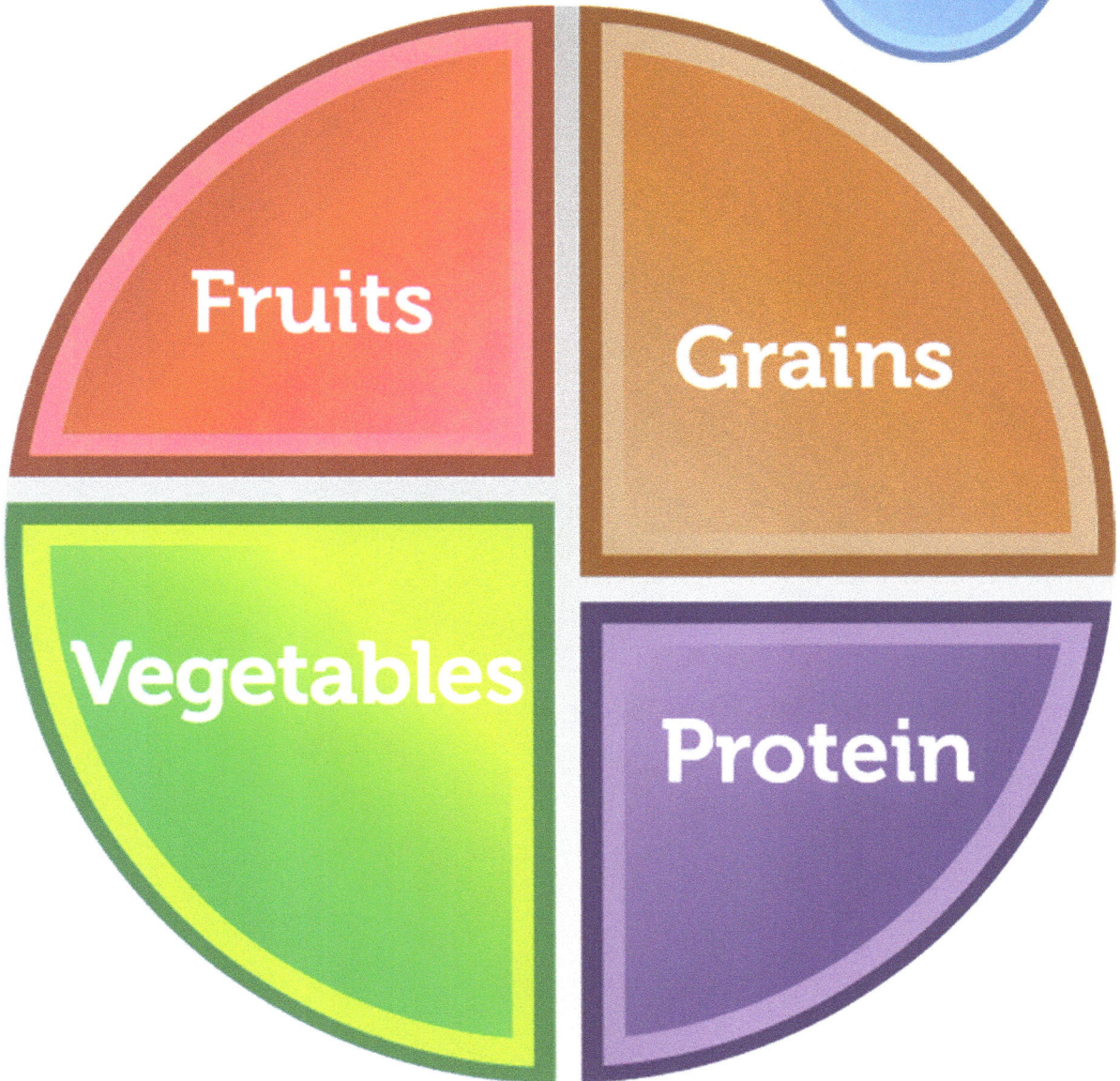

FACE 1

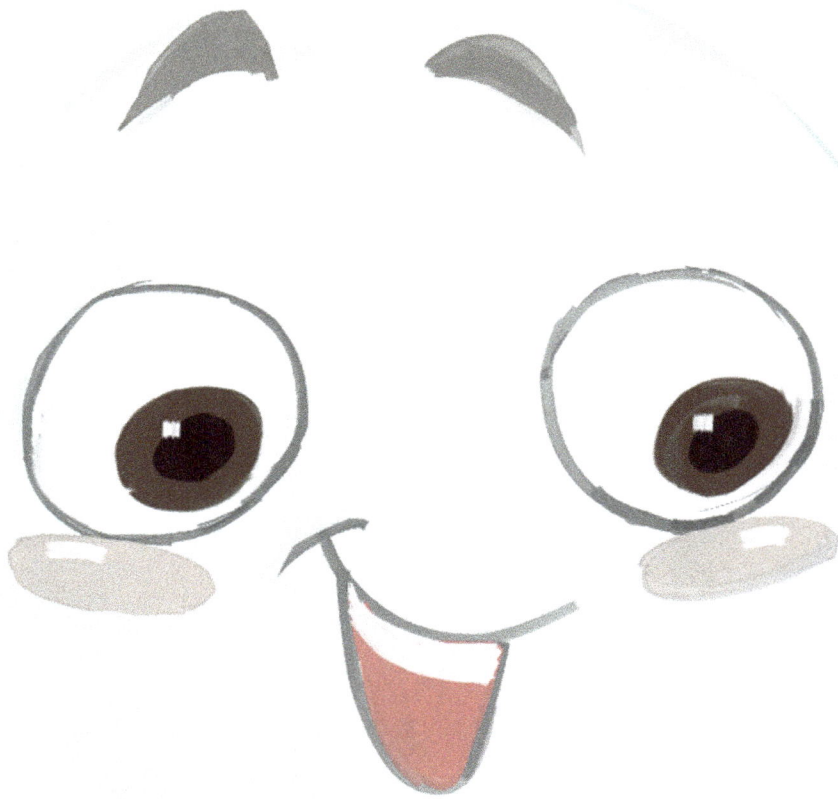

FACE 2

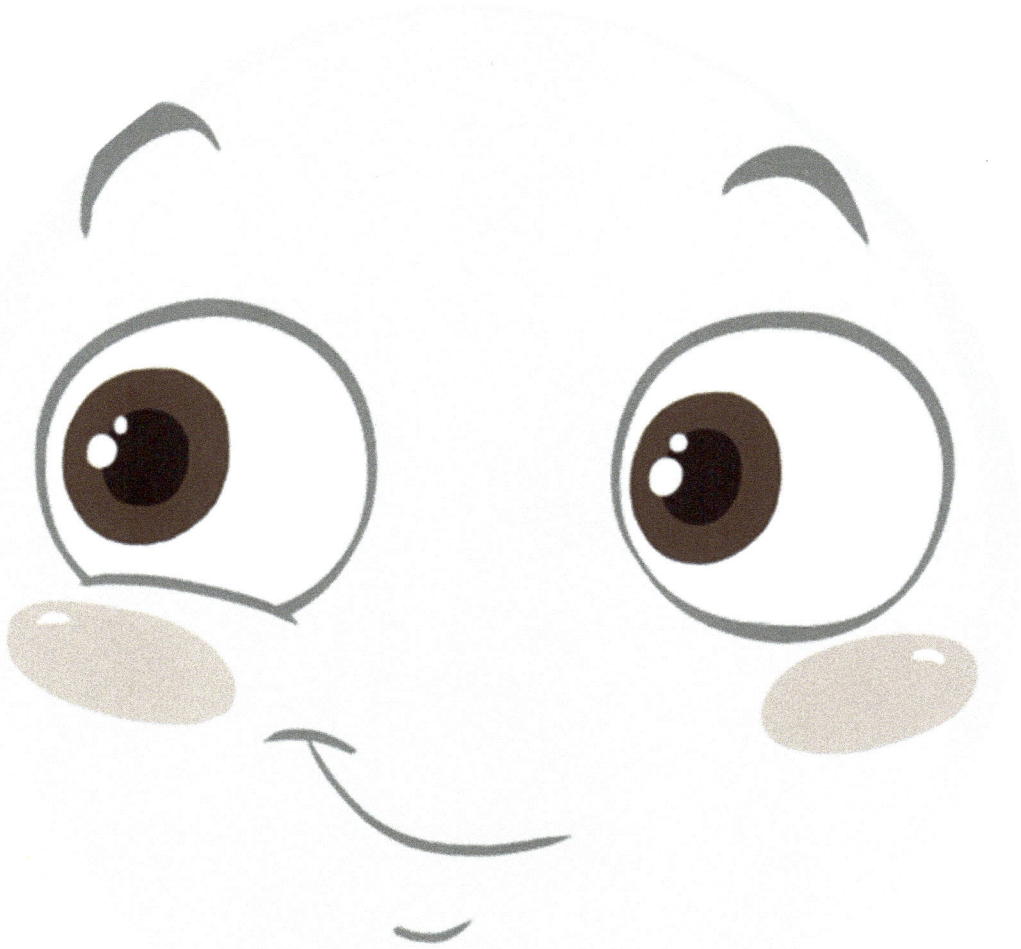

FACE 3

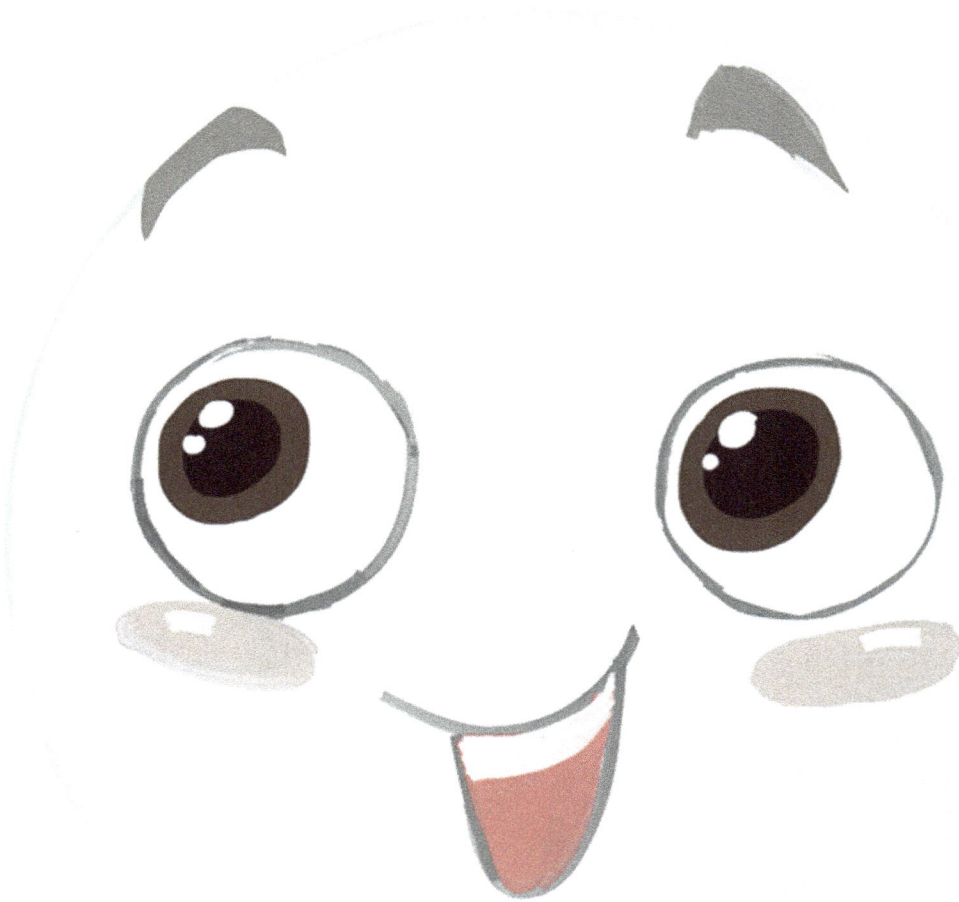

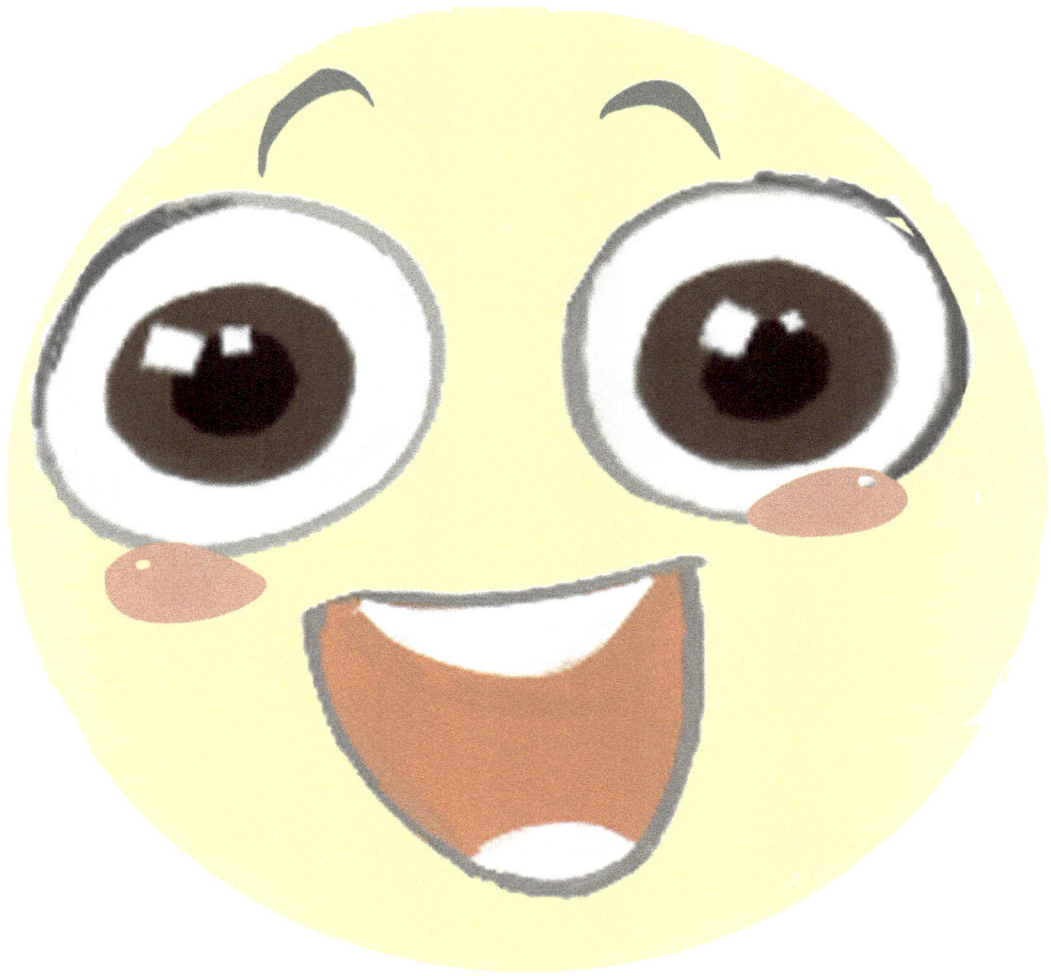

FACE 5

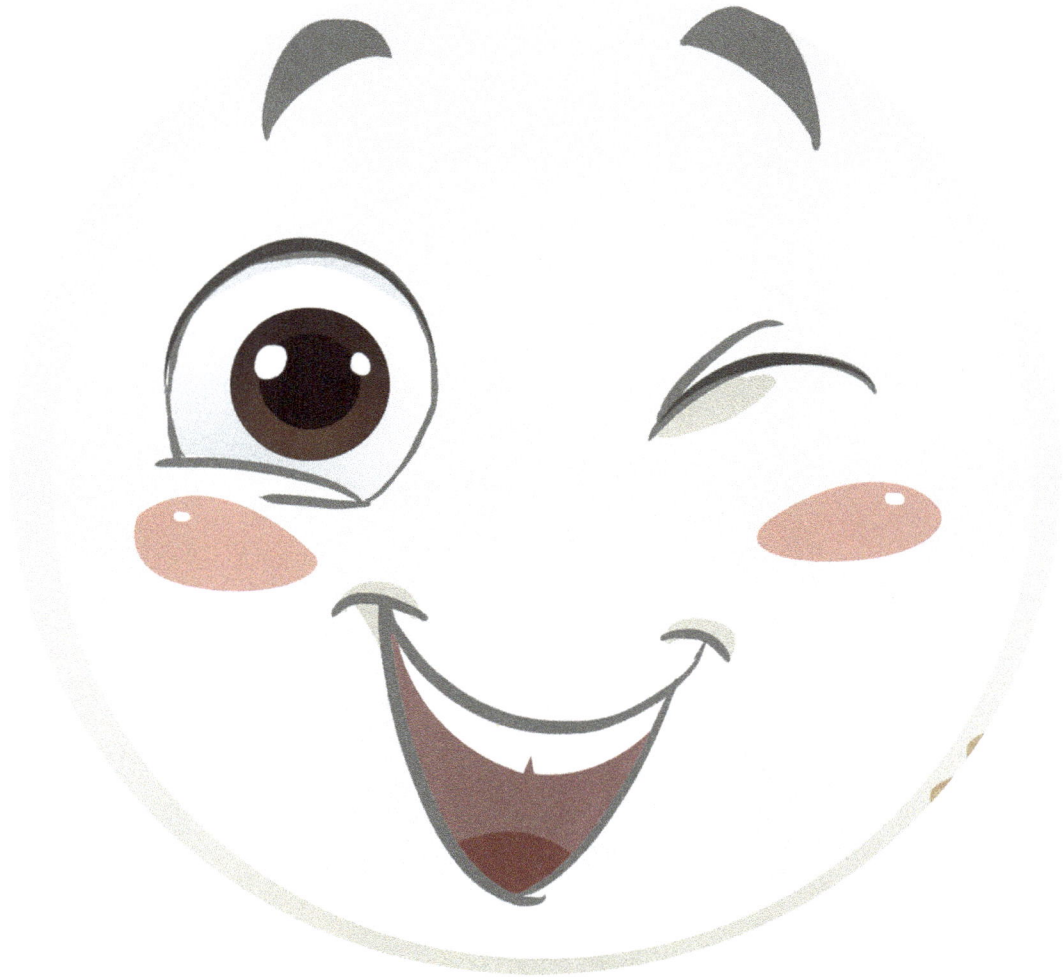

LEFT ARMS

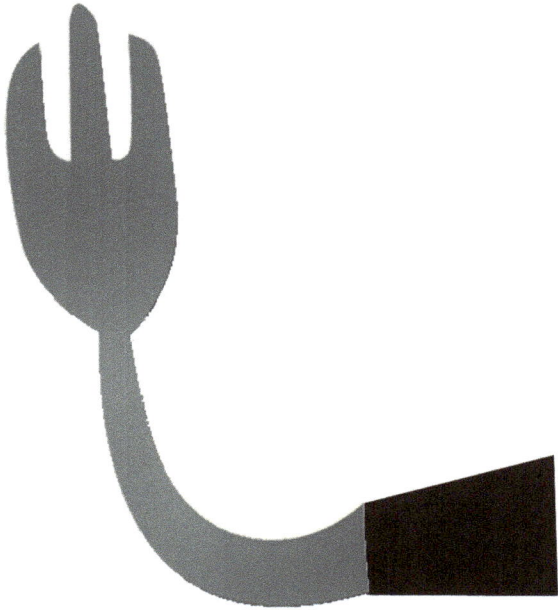

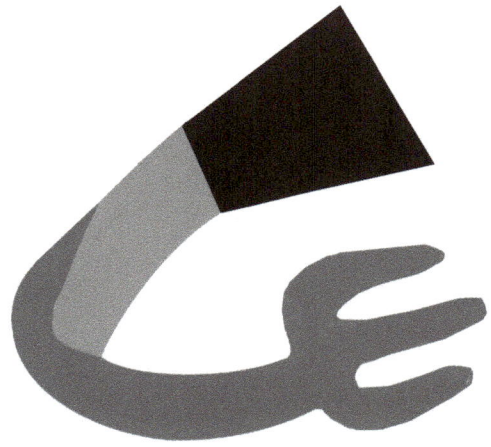

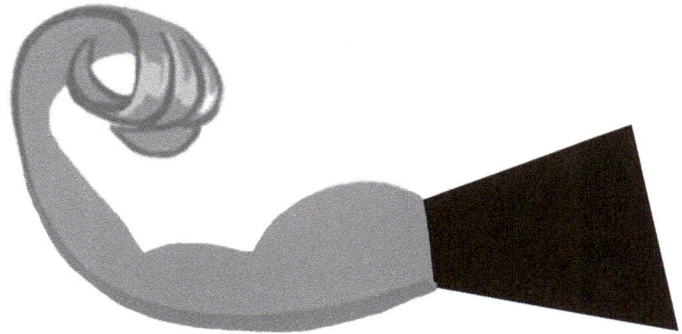

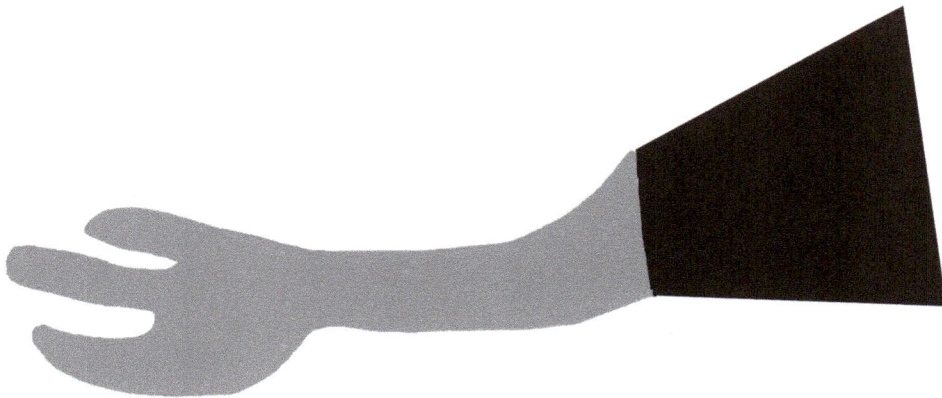

LEFT ARMS

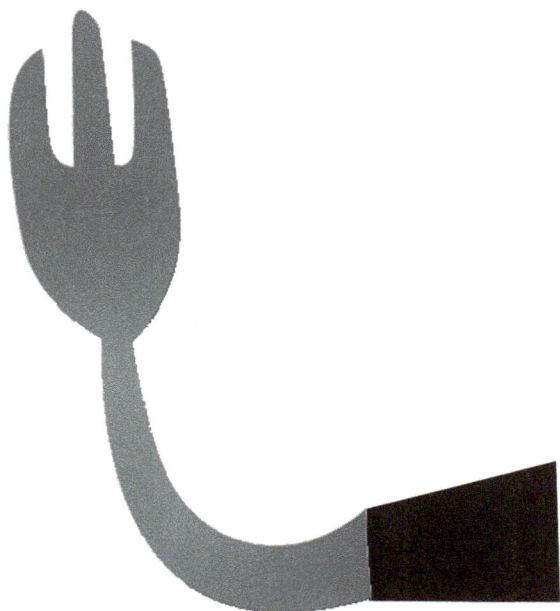
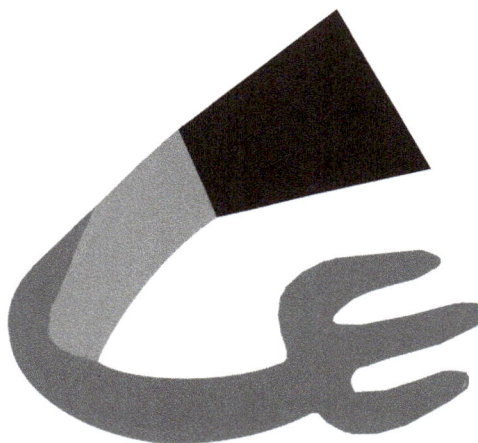
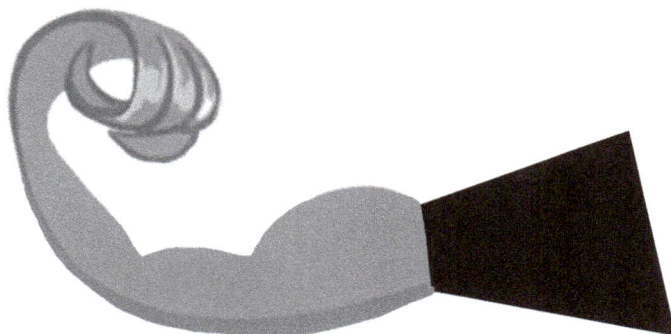
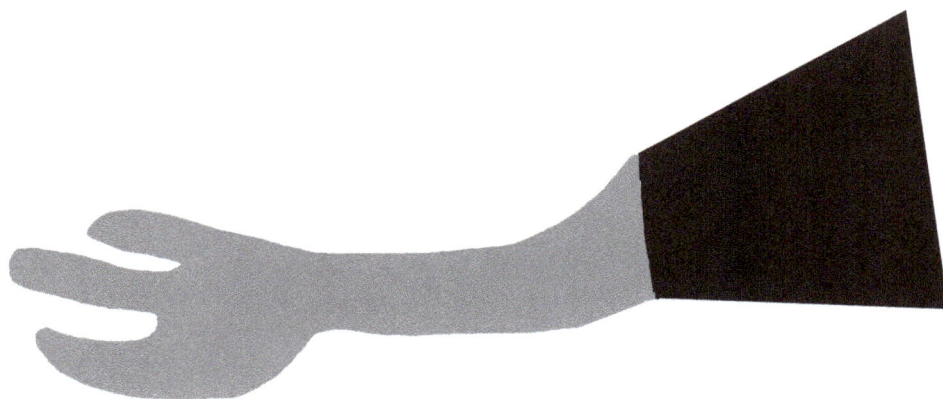

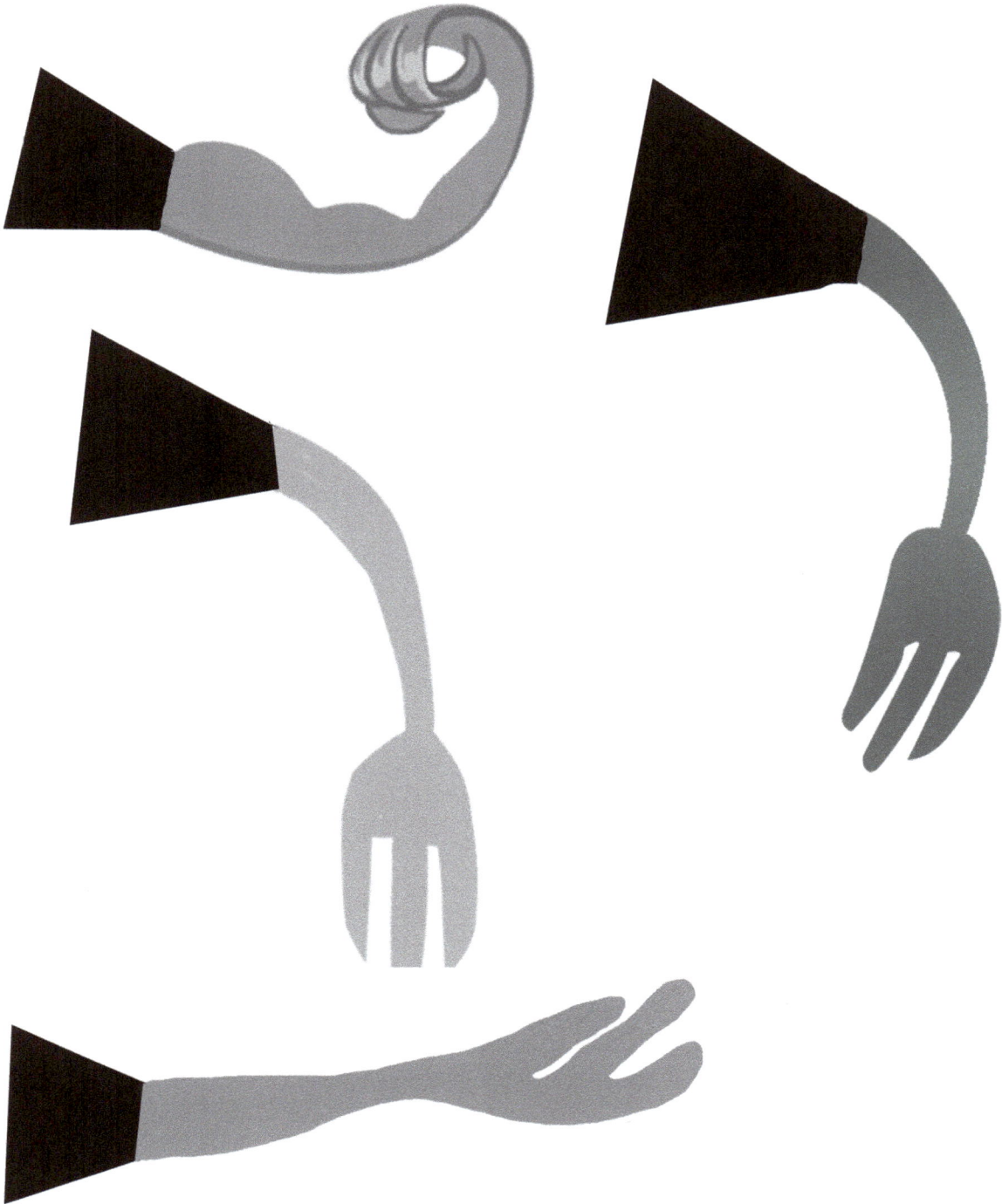

RIGHT ARMS

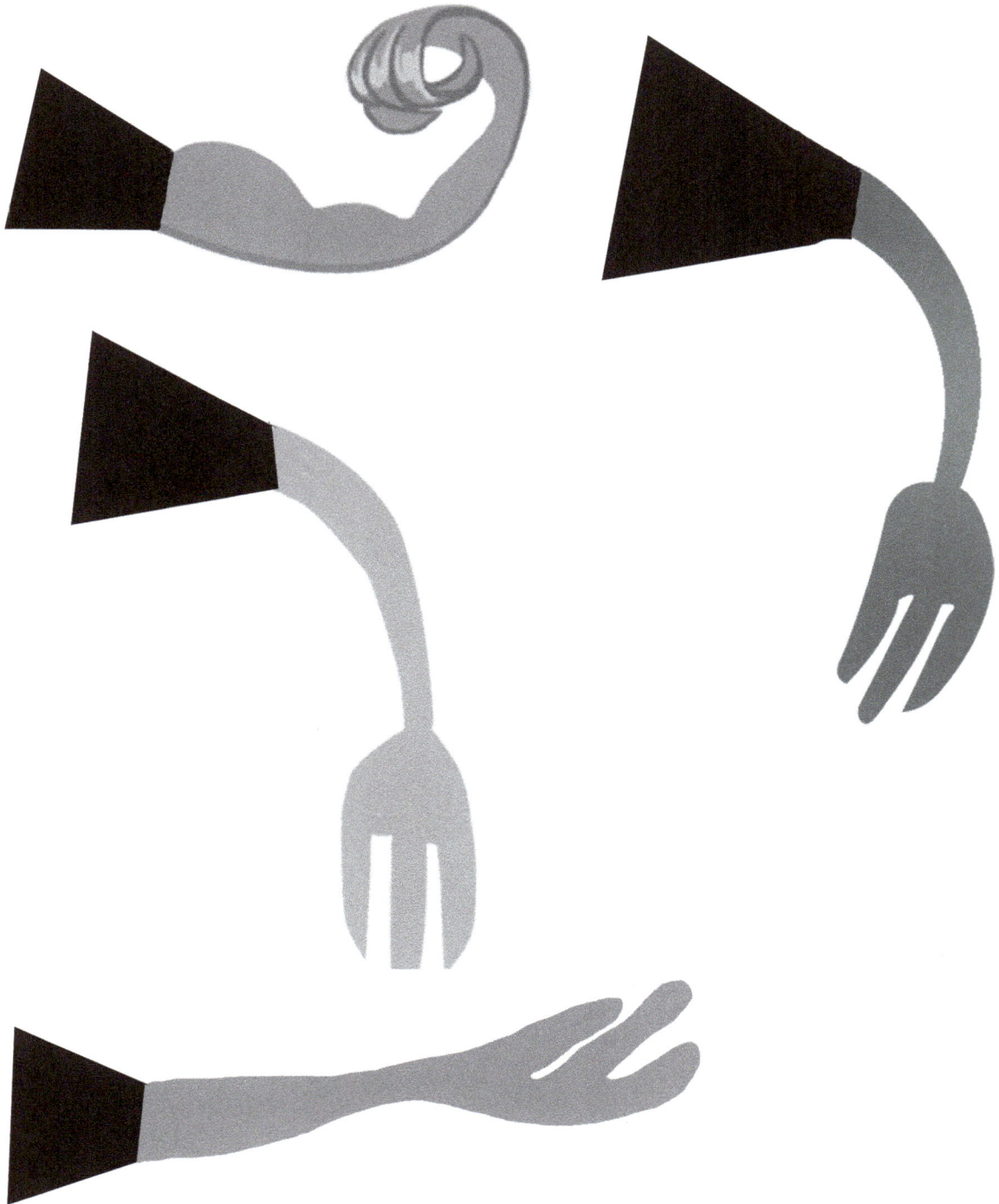

RIGHT ARMS

Legs

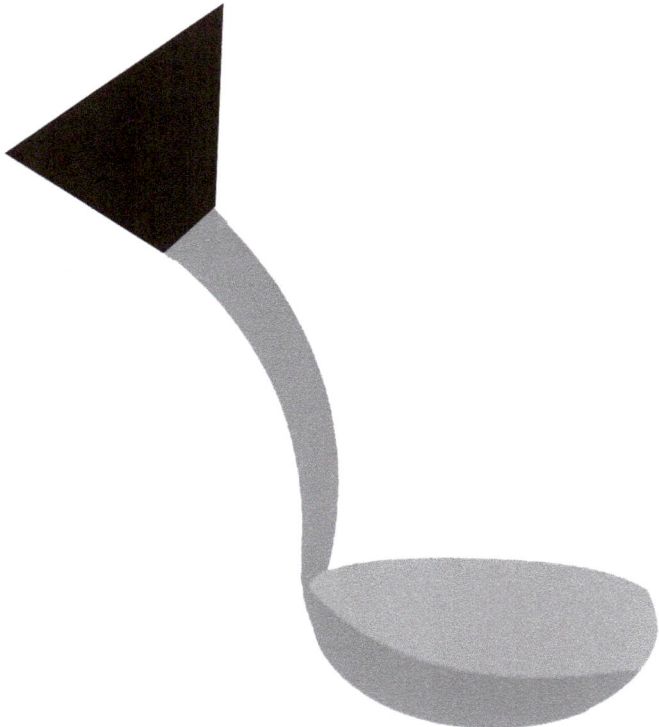
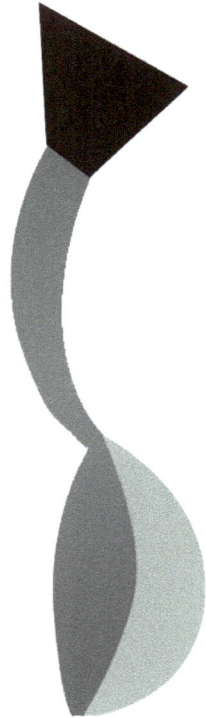
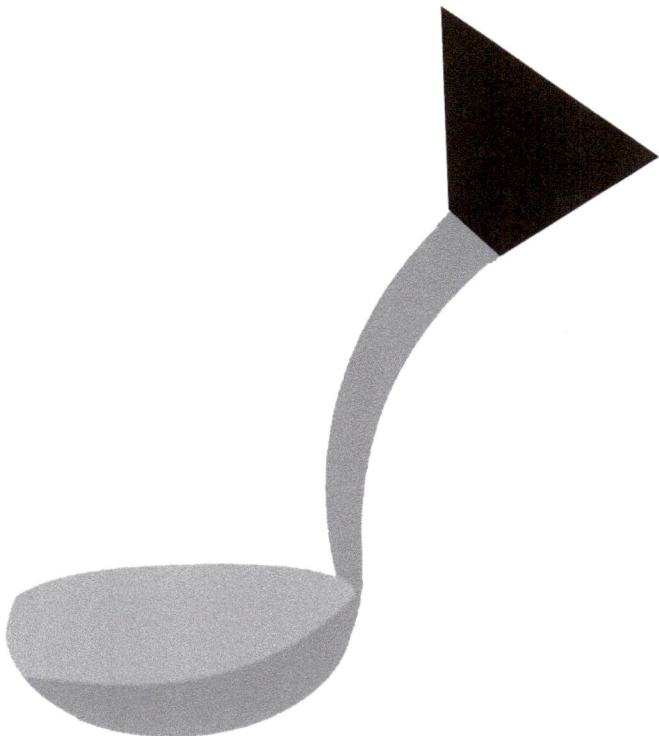
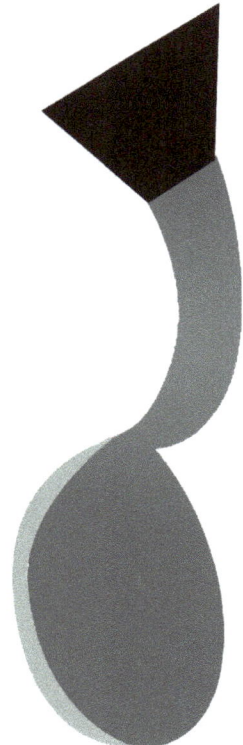

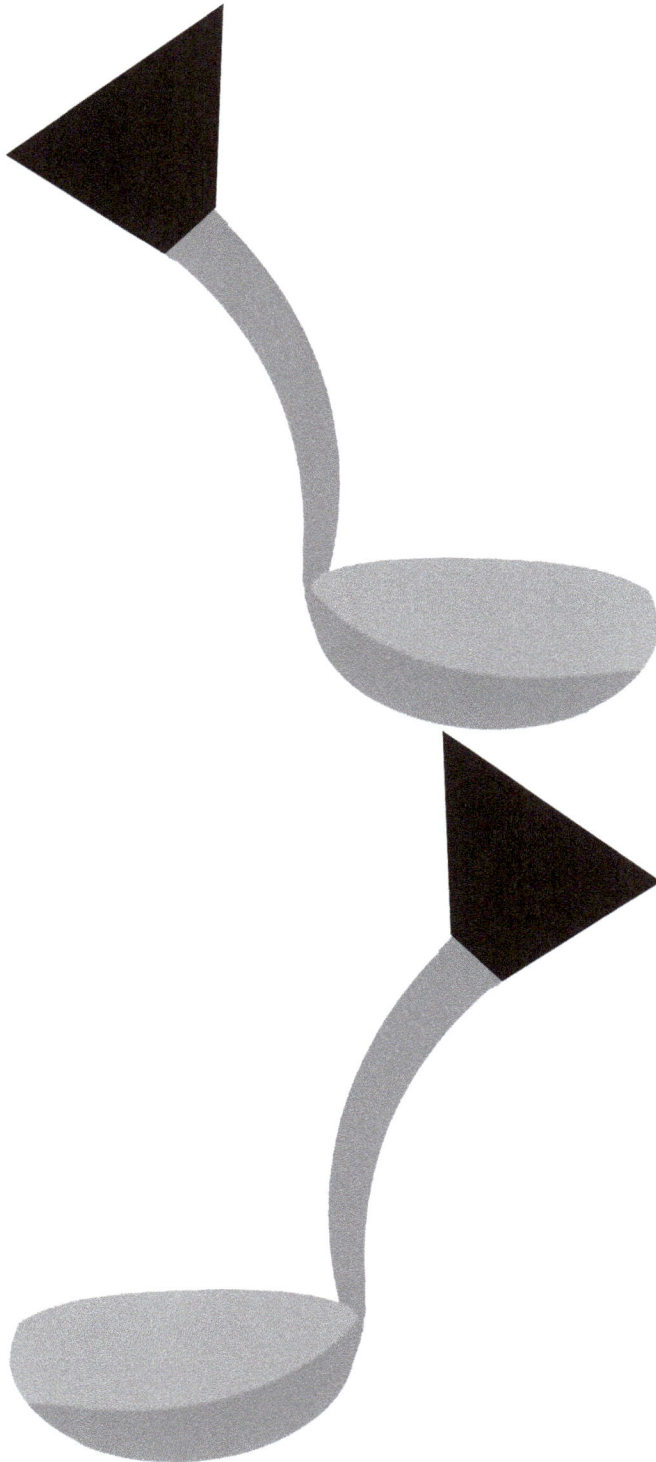

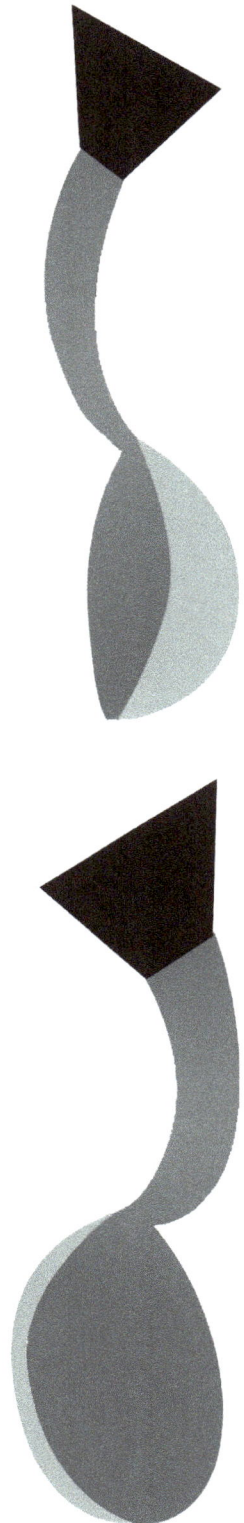

Legs

75

SUPER-NATURAL POWER FOOD GROUPS

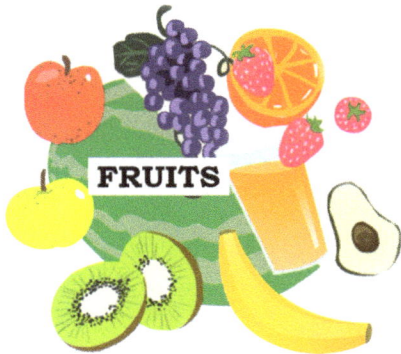

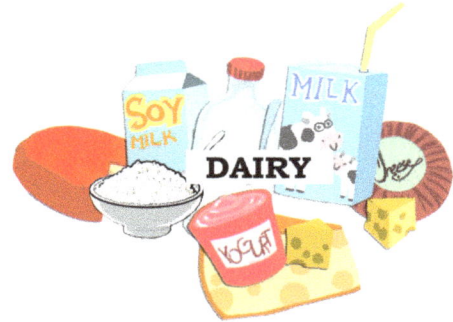

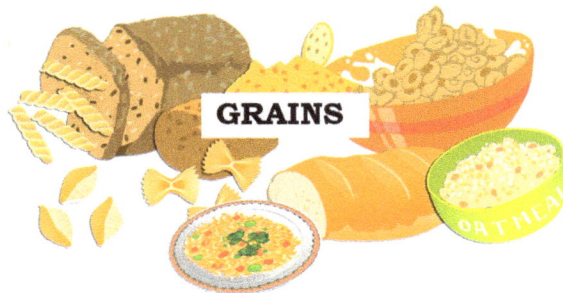

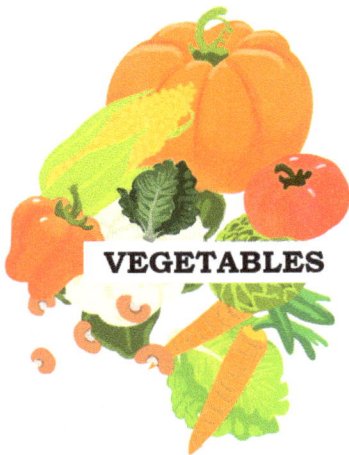

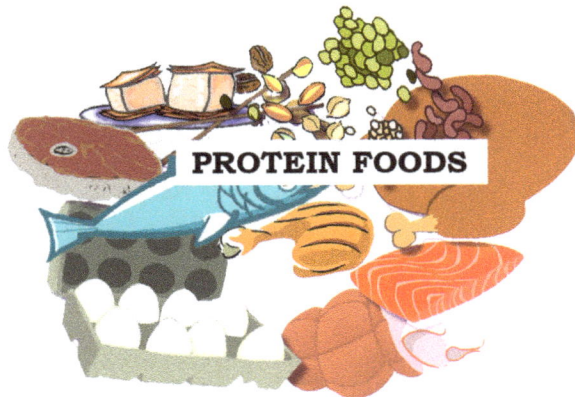

FRUITS

DAIRY

GRAINS

VEGETABLES

PROTEIN FOODS

SUPER-NATURAL POWER FOOD GROUPS

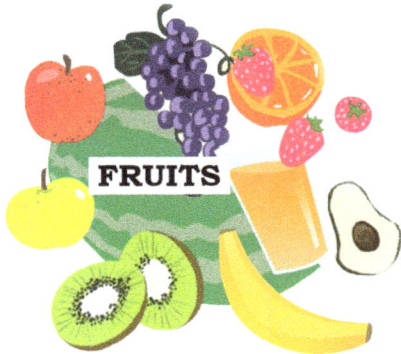

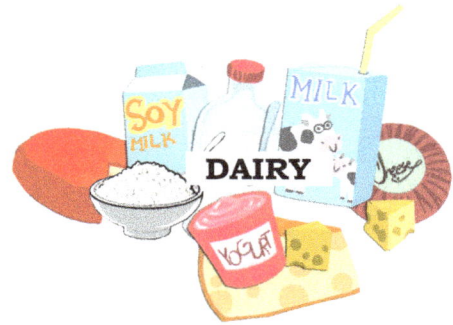

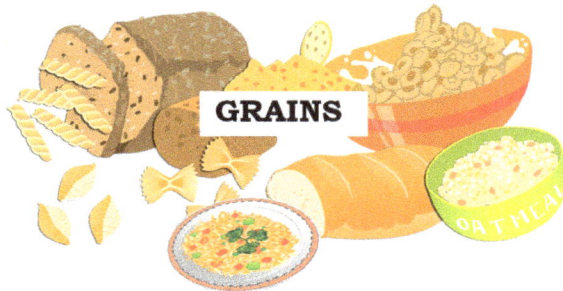

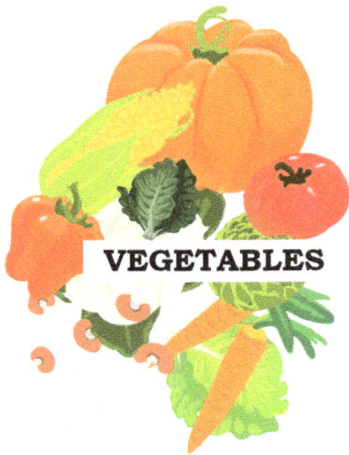

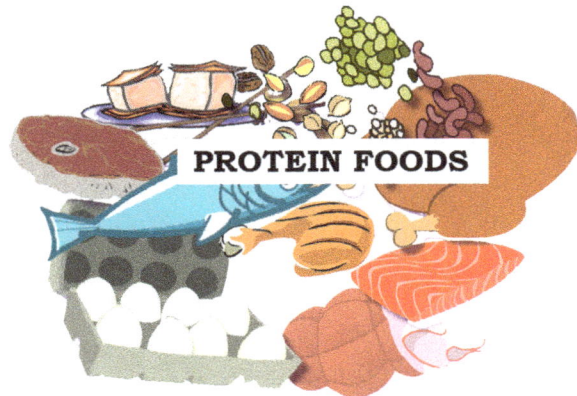

FRUITS

DAIRY

GRAINS

VEGETABLES

PROTEIN FOODS

SUPER-NATURAL
POWER FOOD GROUPS

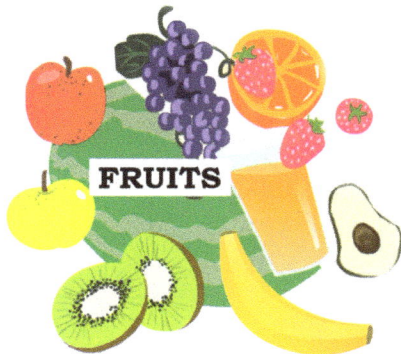

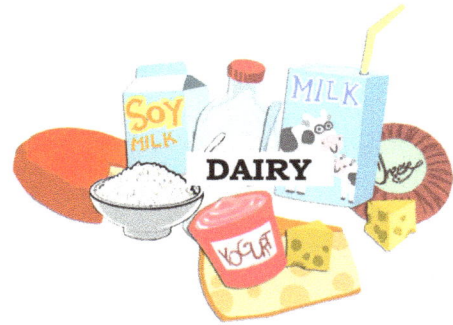

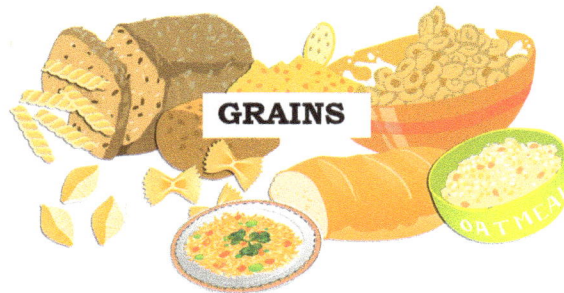

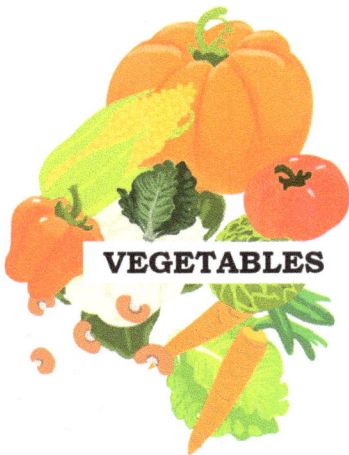

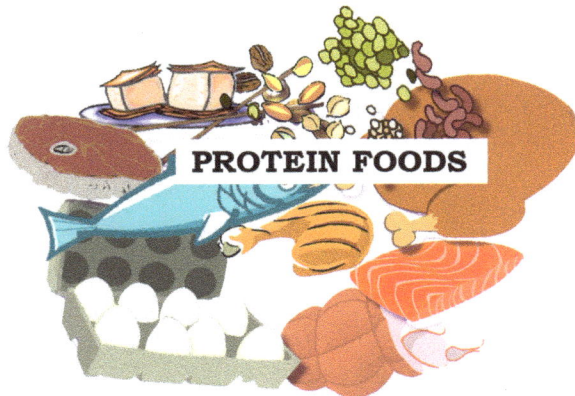

FRUITS

DAIRY

GRAINS

VEGETABLES

PROTEIN FOODS

MORE ABOUT PROTEIN FOODS

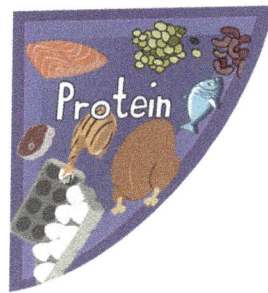

Protein foods help to build strong muscles, bones, skin, blood, and other body parts. They also help us have energy so we don't get tired quickly.

Protein foods can come from animals or plants.

Some examples of animal protein foods are chicken, turkey, fish, beef, ham, and eggs. It's best to eat animal protein foods that are not fatty, except for fish. Fatty fish such as salmon, trout, sardines, anchovies, herring, certain oysters, and certain mackerel contain particular oils that give us extra special health benefits.

Foods such as dried beans, lentils, chickpeas, nuts, and tofu, are examples of protein foods from plants.

Each kind of protein food has its own special way of keeping us healthy, so it's important to eat all different kinds of protein foods.

COMMONLY EATEN PROTEIN FOODS *

TIP: To find out the healthiest portion sizes for protein foods and how many portions to eat each day, visit ChooseMyPlate.gov.

Meats

Lean cuts of:

beef

ham

lamb

pork

veal

Game Meats:

bison

rabbit

venison

Lean Ground Meats:

beef

pork

lamb

Lean Luncheon or Deli meats

Organ Meats:

liver

giblets

Processed Soy Products

tofu
(bean curd made from soybeans)

veggie burgers

tempeh

textured vegetable protein (TVP)

Eggs

chicken eggs

duck eggs

Beans and Peas

bean burgers

black beans

black-eyed peas

chickpeas
(garbanzo beans)

falafel

kidney beans

lentils

lima beans (mature)

navy beans

pinto beans

soy beans

split peas

white beans

COMMONLY EATEN PROTEIN FOODS *

*Adapted from the USDA Center for Nutrition Policy and Promotion's ChooseMyPlate.gov website.

Nuts and Seeds

almonds

cashews

hazelnuts (filberts)

mixed nuts

peanuts

peanut butter

pecans

pistachios

pumpkin seeds

sesame seeds

sunflower seeds

walnuts

Seafood

Finfish:

catfish

cod

flounder

haddock

halibut

herring

mackerel

salmon

sea bass

snapper

swordfish

pollock

porgy

trout

tuna

Seafood (continued)

Shellfish:

clams

crab

crayfish

lobster

mussels

octopus

oysters

scallops

squid (calamari)

shrimp

Canned fish:

anchovies

clams

tuna

sardines

MORE ABOUT FRUITS AND VEGETABLES

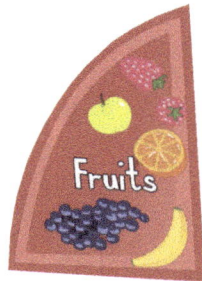

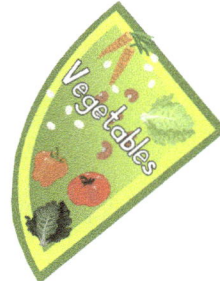

Eating a variety of fruits and vegetables helps to protect our bodies from disease, and keeps our bodies healthy.

Fruits and vegetables come from plants and can be found in many wonderful colors. Some examples are broccoli (green), bananas (white), sweet potatoes (yellow/orange), and raisins (blue/purple). What other examples can you give?

Each fruit and vegetable plays its own role in keeping us healthy. Therefore, it's very important to eat many different kinds of fruits and vegetables in order to be as healthy as possible and to protect our bodies from disease.

It's best to eat whole, fresh fruits. If eating canned fruits or fruit juices, choose those that have no added sugar.

Try to eat whole, fresh vegetables. If eating frozen or canned vegetables, it's best to choose those with little or no added salt.

You can find out whether a food has added salt and/or sugar by reading the ingredients label.

Beans and peas, which are part of the protein foods group, are also part of the vegetable group, because they provide many of the same kinds of health benefits that vegetables do.

COMMONLY EATEN FRUITS *

TIP: To find out the healthiest portion sizes for fruits and how many portions of fruits to eat each day, visit ChooseMyPlate.gov.

*Adapted from the USDA Center for Nutrition Policy and Promotion's ChooseMyPlate.gov website.

Fruits
apples

apricots

bananas

cherries

grapefruit

grapes

kiwi fruit

lemons

limes

mangoes

nectarines

oranges

peaches

pears

papaya

pineapple

plums

prunes

raisins

tangerines

Berries
strawberries

blueberries

raspberries

Melons
cantaloupe

honeydew

watermelon

Mixed fruits
fruit cocktail

100% Fruit juice
orange

apple

grape

grapefruit

COMMONLY EATEN VEGETABLES *

TIP: To find out the healthiest portion sizes for vegetables and how many portions to eat each day, visit ChooseMyPlate.gov.

Dark green vegetables

bok choy

broccoli

collard greens

dark green leafy lettuce

kale

mesclun

mustard greens

romaine lettuce

spinach

turnip greens

watercress

Starchy vegetables

cassava

corn

fresh cowpeas, field peas, or black-eyed peas (not dry)

green bananas

green peas

green lima beans

Starchy vegetables (continued)

plantains

potatoes

taro

water chestnuts

Red & orange vegetables

acorn squash

butternut squash

carrots

hubbard squash

pumpkin

red peppers

sweet potatoes

tomatoes

tomato juice

Beans and peas

black beans

black-eyed peas (mature, dry)

garbanzo beans (chickpeas)

kidney beans

lentils

COMMONLY EATEN VEGETABLES *

*Adapted from the USDA Center for Nutrition Policy and Promotion's ChooseMyPlate.gov website.

Beans and peas (continued)

navy beans

pinto beans

soy beans

split peas

white beans

Other vegetables

artichokes

asparagus

avocado

bean sprouts

beets

brussels sprouts

cabbage

cauliflower

celery

cucumbers

eggplant

green beans

green peppers

iceberg (head) lettuce

Other vegetables (continued)

mushrooms

okra

onions

turnips

wax beans

zucchini

MORE ABOUT DAIRY FOODS

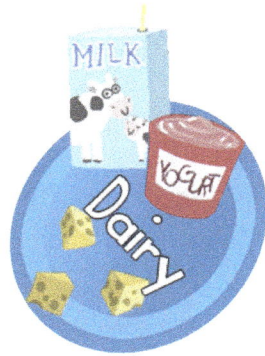

Dairy foods are foods that are made from milk. Dairy foods contain calcium, which helps to build strong bones. We also need dairy foods to help our bodies in other ways.

Fat-free and low-fat dairy foods are healthier than whole-fat dairy foods.

If you find it difficult to digest dairy foods, try eating smaller portions. There are also lactose-free and lower-lactose milk products available. These include lactose-reduced or lactose-free milk, yogurt, and cheese, and calcium-fortified soymilk (soy beverage).

Some non-dairy foods can be good sources of calcium if eaten in sufficient amounts. These include soybeans, tofu, spinach, broccoli, collards, kale, mustard greens, turnip greens and bok choy.

Foods and beverages with added calcium such as cereals, orange juice, or rice or almond beverages may provide calcium, but may not provide the other nutrients found in dairy products.

It's best to choose dairy products that have no added sugar. How can you tell? Read the ingredients label.

COMMONLY EATEN DAIRY FOODS AND DAIRY PRODUCTS *

TIP: To find out the healthiest portion sizes for dairy products and how many portions to eat each day, visit ChooseMyPlate.gov.

*Adapted from the USDA Center for Nutrition Policy and Promotion's ChooseMyPlate.gov website.

Milk

All fluid milk:

  fat-free (skim)

  low-fat (1%)

  reduced-fat (2%)

  whole-fat

  lactose-reduced milks

  lactose-free milks

Flavored milks:

  chocolate

  strawberry

Milk-based desserts

puddings

ice milk

frozen yogurt

ice cream

Calcium-fortified soymilk (soy beverage)

Cheese

Hard natural cheeses:

  cheddar

  mozzarella

  swiss

  parmesan

Soft cheeses:

  ricotta

  cottage cheese

Processed cheeses:

  american

Yogurt

All yogurt:

  fat-free

  low-fat

  reduced-fat

  whole-fat

MORE ABOUT GRAINS

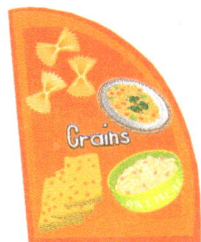

Take a peek inside
a grain kernel....

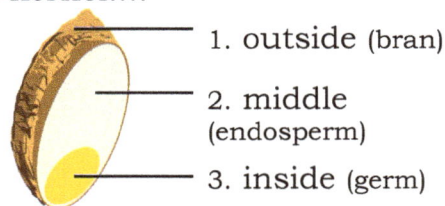

1. outside (bran)

2. middle (endosperm)

3. inside (germ)

Grains come from plants such as wheat, rice, corn, and others. Grain foods are made from the kernels of a grain plant. Some examples of these foods are bread, rice, cereal, and pasta.

There are three parts to the kernel of a grain plant; the outside, the middle, and the inside. The outside helps to keep our tummies healthy. The middle part gives us energy. The inside helps to protect our health. Since each part contains important nutrients, it's best to eat foods made with all three parts.

Foods that have all three parts are called *whole grain* foods. Whole grain foods are healthier than foods made from only part of the kernel. At least half of the grain foods we eat should be from whole grain foods, so we can be as healthy as possible.

Foods that don't have all three kernel parts are called refined grains.

Some examples of popular whole grain foods include whole wheat bread, whole wheat pasta, brown rice, popcorn, and oatmeal.

To find out whether a food is made from the whole of the grain kernel, check the first few ingredients listed for words such as "whole grain" or "whole wheat". Some foods are made from a mixture of whole and refined grains.

COMMONLY EATEN GRAINS AND GRAIN PRODUCTS *

TIP: To find out the healthiest portion sizes for grain products and how many portions to eat each day, visit ChooseMyPlate.gov.

TIP: Find whole grain choices fast by choosing products that have the Whole Grain Stamp (see below). Learn more at wholegrainscouncil.org.

TIP: Some foods contain a mixture of whole grains and refined grains. Choose foods that have the word "whole" at the beginning of the ingredients label.

Adapted from the USDA Center for Nutrition Policy and Promotion's ChooseMyPlate.gov website.

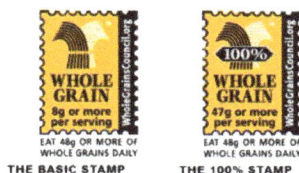

Whole Grain Stamp

Whole Grains

amaranth

brown rice

buckwheat

bulgur (cracked wheat)

millet

oatmeal

popcorn

rolled oats

quinoa

sorghum

triticale

whole grain barley

whole grain cornmeal

whole rye

whole wheat bread

whole wheat crackers

Whole Grains
(continued)

whole wheat pasta

whole wheat sandwich buns and rolls

whole wheat tortillas

wild rice

Ready-to-eat breakfast cereals, such as:

 whole grain cereals

 muesli

Refined Grains

cornbread

corn tortillas

Refined Grains
(continued)

couscous

crackers

flour tortillas

grits

noodles

pitas

pretzels

white bread

white sandwich buns and rolls

white rice

Pastas, such as:

 spaghetti

 macaroni

Ready-to-eat breakfast cereals, such as:

 corn flakes

MORE ABOUT OILS *

Oils are fats that are liquid at room temperature. The healthiest oils are those from vegetables, nuts, seeds, olives, avocados, and some fish. Avocados are part of the fruit group, but they are also a good source of healthy oil.

Oils are not a food group, but because they contain some essential nutrients, oils are part of a healthy eating plan. Oils are very high in calories, so we limit the amount we eat. Learn more at ChooseMyPlate.gov.

TIP: To find out the healthiest portion sizes for oils and how many portions to eat each day, visit ChooseMyPlate.gov.

*Adapted from the USDA Center for Nutrition Policy and Promotion's ChooseMyPlate.gov website.

Commonly eaten oils:

canola oil

corn oil

cottonseed oil

olive oil

safflower oil

soybean oil

sunflower oil

Foods high in oils:

nuts

olives

some fish

avocados

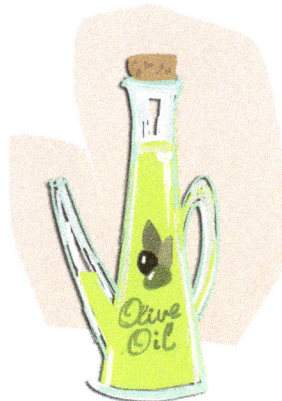

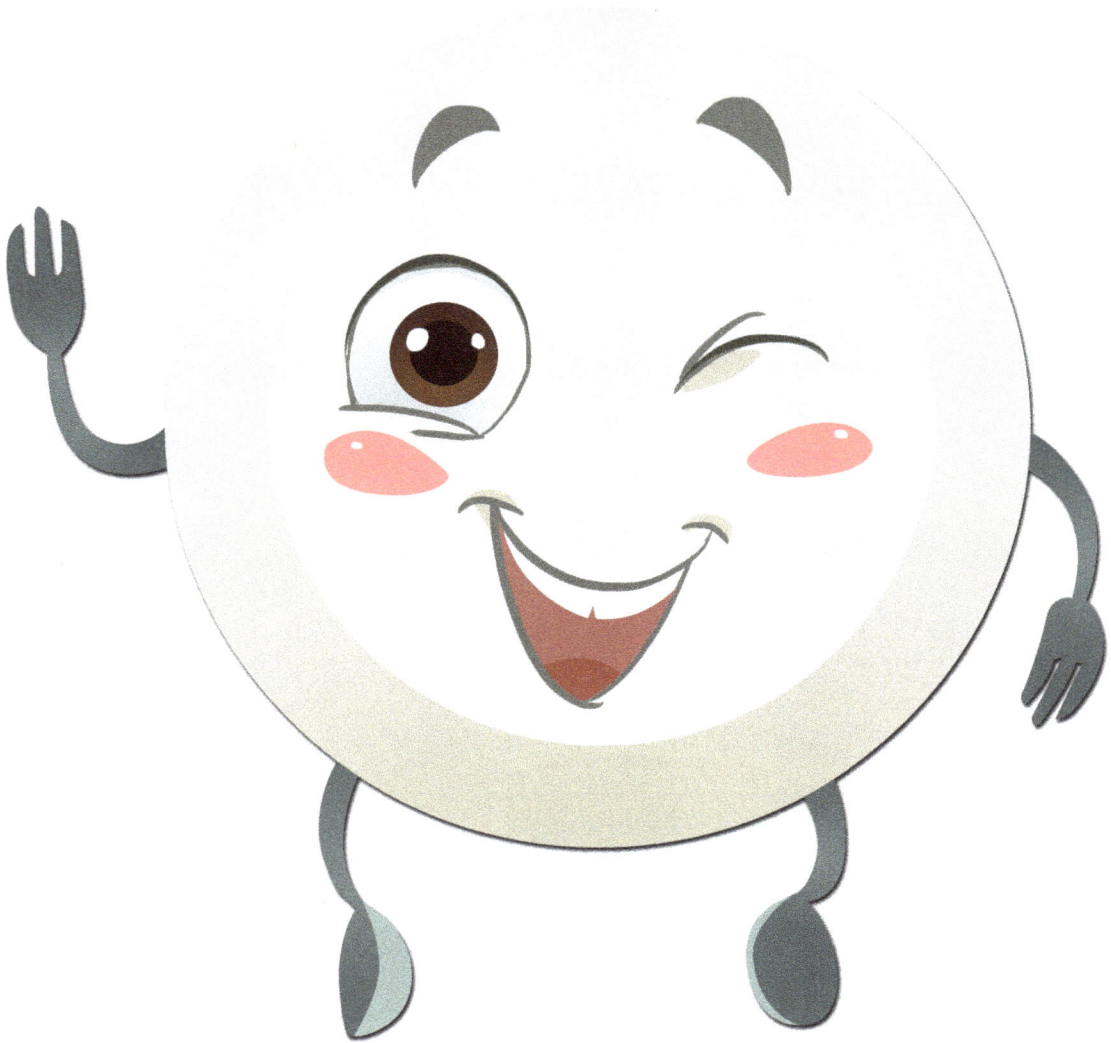

ACKNOWLEDGEMENTS

First, a most special thank you to Christina Krati, the wonderful illustrator of this book, for taking this fabulous journey with me, and for translating my vision into something everyone can see.

Along the way, many individuals kept me company with their invaluable honesty, encouragement, suggestions, and support.

To Joyce A., Naomi B., Steven D., Jennifer L., Lori C., Debbie D., Mollie F., Laurie H., Dena H., Yael K. and family, Cheryl L., Alexa L., Janie L., and Eileen S., and most especially Dana Z.: Thank you all so very much!

Many special thanks as well to my colleagues Connie Evers, MS, RDN, LD, and Nancy Mazarin, MS, RDN, CDN, CNS, for their wisdom and insight.

To my wonderful children, Randon and Erin, and my incredible family: Thank you so much for sharing my dream, and for your unlimited patience and support during this lengthy and challenging, but thoroughly enjoyable, creative binge!

And, to my David, for *always* believing in me,
and *always* encouraging me to be the best I can be!

ABOUT THE AUTHOR

Donna Daun Lester, MA, RDN, CDN, is a Registered Dietitian Nutritionist, Certified Dietitian-Nutritionist, and licensed teacher.

Donna has worked as a dietitian-nutritionist in many settings, including private practice, skilled nursing facilities, hospitals, as a Director of Food and Nutrition Services, and as a Nutrition Educator.

After graduating with honors from Queens College, Donna earned a Master of Arts degree in Clinical Nutrition from New York University. The mother of two grown children, Donna lives with her husband on Long Island, in New York.

ABOUT THE ILLUSTRATOR

Originally from Greece, Christina Krati holds a Bachelor of Fine Arts degree in Graphic Design from the Technological Educational Institute (T.E.I.) of Athens, Greece.

An accomplished designer, artist and illustrator, Christina now resides in New York, New York.

www.ingramcontent.com/pod-product-compliance
Lightning Source LLC
Chambersburg PA
CBHW050106220326
41598CB00043B/7401